Artificial and Cognitive Computing for Sustainable Healthcare Systems in Smart Cities

International Perspectives in Decision Analytics and Operations Research Set
coordinated by
Prasenjit Chatterjee

Volume 3

Artificial and Cognitive Computing for Sustainable Healthcare Systems in Smart Cities

Edited by

Devasis Pradhan
Prasanna Kumar Sahu
Hla Myo Tun
Prasenjit Chatterjee

iSTE

WILEY

First published 2024 in Great Britain and the United States by ISTE Ltd and John Wiley & Sons, Inc.

ISTE Ltd
27-37 St George's Road
London SW19 4EU
UK

www.iste.co.uk

John Wiley & Sons, Inc.
111 River Street
Hoboken, NJ 07030
USA

www.wiley.com

Library of Congress Control Number: 2023951338

British Library Cataloguing-in-Publication Data
A CIP record for this book is available from the British Library
ISBN 978-1-78630-864-1

Contents

Preface

Welcome to the intriguing world of "Artificial and Cognitive Computing for Sustainable Healthcare Systems in Smart Cities". In an era where our lives are becoming increasingly entwined with technology, the fusion of artificial intelligence and cognitive computing with healthcare in the context of smart cities represents a groundbreaking frontier. This preface sets the stage for a compelling journey through the pages of this book, which explores the transformative potential of these cutting-edge technologies for the betterment of healthcare systems in urban environments.

Smart cities are on the rise, and with their rapid urbanization come a unique set of challenges and opportunities. These urban centers are harnessing the power of data, connectivity and intelligent systems to enhance the quality of life for their citizens. One of the most critical domains where this transformation is taking place is healthcare. The demand for efficient, sustainable and patient-centric healthcare services is escalating in tandem with urban growth, and this book explores how artificial and cognitive computing can serve as catalysts for positive change.

In this book, you will find a comprehensive exploration of the fusion of artificial intelligence, machine learning and cognitive computing with healthcare systems. We bring together experts and thought leaders from various fields to share their insights and experiences. Their contributions offer diverse perspectives on the challenges and potential solutions in the realm of sustainable healthcare within smart cities. As you navigate through these chapters, you will gain a brief understanding of how AI-driven systems can be leveraged to mitigate healthcare disparities, promote

---

Chapter written by Devasis PRADHAN and Prasanna Kumar SAHU.

preventive care, and create more resilient healthcare infrastructures in urban environments.

The topics covered within these pages include the ethical considerations of AI in healthcare, the implementation of IoT devices, the development of data-driven healthcare policies and the human-centered design of smart city healthcare services. Our aim is to inspire and equip readers to harness the potential of these technologies for creating sustainable, accessible and efficient healthcare systems that cater to the needs of a rapidly urbanizing world. We hope that this book fosters a deeper appreciation of the exciting possibilities that lie ahead and empower you to be an active participant in the journey towards a future where healthcare in smart cities is not only intelligent but also deeply compassionate.

Thank you for embarking on this intellectual journey with us. We invite you to continue reading to explore the transformative world of "Artificial and Cognitive Computing for Sustainable Healthcare Systems in Smart Cities".

January 2024

Introduction

In the 21st century, the world is undergoing an unprecedented transformation. Our cities are evolving into smart, connected ecosystems, where data flows like the lifeblood of urban existence. As these urban centers swell with population and complexity, so do the challenges they face, particularly in the realm of healthcare. The need for sustainable, efficient and accessible healthcare systems in smart cities has never been more pressing. It is in this context that we embark on a journey of discovery in "Artificial and Cognitive Computing for Sustainable Healthcare Systems in Smart Cities". Smart cities represent the nexus of technological innovation, urbanization and the ever-evolving field of healthcare. These cities are not merely clusters of buildings and streets, but intricate networks of data and technology, designed to enhance the quality of life for their residents. At the heart of this transformation lies the intersection of artificial intelligence and cognitive computing with healthcare; a convergence that promises to revolutionize the way we receive, access and experience healthcare services.

This book is your portal into this exciting and dynamic world. In the pages that follow, we will explore the profound impact of artificial intelligence (AI) and cognitive computing on the healthcare landscape within smart cities. We will delve into the realms of data analytics, machine learning and advanced algorithms to understand how these technologies are changing the way healthcare is delivered, managed and experienced by patients. Our exploration encompasses the full spectrum of healthcare, from diagnostics to treatment, from patient records to population health management. We recognize that the implementation of artificial and cognitive computing in healthcare is not without its challenges. Ethical

Chapter written by Devasis PRADHAN, Prasanna Kumar SAHU, Hla Myo TUN and Prasenjit CHATTERJEE.

considerations, data security and the need to ensure equitable access to healthcare services are integral to this discussion. In these pages, we will scrutinize these vital issues, providing a well-rounded perspective on the complex interplay between technology and humanity.

This book serves as a comprehensive guide for healthcare professionals, policymakers, technologists, researchers and anyone intrigued by the potential of AI and cognitive computing in the healthcare sector. It is a resource that equips you with the knowledge and insights required to navigate the ever-evolving landscape of healthcare in smart cities. As we journey through the chapters ahead, we invite you to ponder the possibilities and implications of artificial and cognitive computing for healthcare in smart cities. This is a realm where technology not only meets human needs but anticipates them, where cities are not only smart but also compassionate, and where healthcare is not just a service but a right.

Join us as we embark on a transformative exploration of "Artificial and Cognitive Computing for Sustainable Healthcare Systems in Smart Cities". Together, let us imagine a future where healthcare is not only a system but also a force for healthier, happier urban living.

1

Artificial Intelligence and its Application in Healthcare Systems

In the current age of contemporary medicine, the healthcare sector has advanced significantly thanks to artificial intelligence (AI) and data science, as well as sophisticated devices and high-end computers. Such AI-assisted health assistance can offer an appraisal of a patient's status, as well as assist clinicians in making key treatment decisions.

As new unique software technologies arise regularly, the FDA has set a goal to implement more stringent regulatory control for these rapidly evolving goods, in order to assure patient safety. Artificial intelligence refers to items that have specific software programs or algorithms that can assess and adapt to new data continually. All are referred to as AI because the technology of the software and the algorithms is very intelligent. It could be determined by how the software is programmed in terms of its ability to analyze statistical data, relying on expert systems that rely on decision trees, their statements and other machine learning techniques. AI algorithms, in essence, are software that learn from fresh data and then act on it. Locked algorithms yield the same result every time the same input is supplied, and they apply the fix function, so some of the examples or techniques have a decision tree or a complex classifier, and those are applied to a given set of inputs. An adjustable algorithm adapts over time in response to new information or data.

The algorithms learn how to change their behavior by adding new input types or new cases to an existing database, and then the new version of the algorithm is deployed in the second phase of the update. Medical device software can be

---

Chapter written by Manthan GHOSH, Deepa DAS, Rohit DEY and Nitish SINHA.
For a color version of all the figures in this chapter, see www.iste.co.uk/pradhan/cognitivecomputing.zip.

expanded using AI, and machine learning technologies again have real-time ability to adapt. Based on real-world feedback, they can improve device performance. When AI- and ML-based programs are incorporated to start treatment, they are then designated as a medical device software.

1.1. History of healthcare system

Modern medicine, or medicine, started to emerge after the Industrial Revolution in the 18th century. Hippocrates is a historical person in medicine. It is closely associated with him and his disciples. History demonstrates how civilizations' attitudes towards sickness have evolved from the prehistoric generation to the recent generation. Babylonian, Chinese, Egyptian and Indian medical traditions are among the earliest.

The microscope was invented as a result of increased understanding during the Renaissance. Humorism was supposed to explain the etiology of disease before the 19th century, but it was progressively supplanted by the germ hypothesis of disease, which led to efficient treatments and even cures for many infectious diseases. Military medics revolutionized trauma care and surgical techniques. The fast rise of cities necessitated the development of public health measures, particularly in the 19th century. Advanced research facilities first appeared in the early 20th century, generally in conjunction with prominent hospitals. Antibiotics were among the novel biological medicines that emerged in the mid-20th century. These advances, together with advances in chemistry, genetics and radiography, resulted in modern medicine. Medicine was significantly professionalized in the 20th century, and new occupations as nurses and physicians opened up for women. One of the first Indian writings dealing with medicine is the Atharvaveda, a sacred Hindu literature originating from the Early Iron Age. The Atharvaveda also has herbal treatments for a variety of diseases. Herbs used to heal diseases would subsequently become an important aspect of Ayurveda. Ayurveda, which means "full wisdom for long life", is another Indian medicinal system. Its two most renowned books are from the Charaka and Sushruta schools of thought. Ayurveda's early roots were constructed on a combination of ancient herbal techniques and a substantial addition of theoretical conceptualizations.

As an alternative form of medicine in India, Unani medicine found deep roots and royal patronage during medieval times. It progressed during the Indian Sultanate and Mughal periods. Unani medicine is very close to Ayurveda. Both are based on the theory of the presence of the elements (in Unani, they are considered to be fire, water, earth and air) in the human body. According to the followers of Unani medicine, these elements are present in different fluids, and their balance leads to health and their imbalance leads to illness.

1.2. Literature studies

Gillies et al. (2016) use AI technology to interpret clinical pictures that include massive amounts of data.

You et al.'s (2018) team investigated how aberrant genetic transcription in lengthy RNAs without coding can be used to identify stomach cancer.

Shin et al. (2010) created an electronic diagnosis optimization approach to locate neurological damage.

Karakülah et al. (2014) used AI technology to identify phenotype information from clinical studies in order to improve the precision of genetic anomaly detection.

Based on a "double-blind validation study", IBM Watson is a trustworthy AI system for supporting cancer detection (Somashekhar et al. 2017).

The benefits of AI have been thoroughly researched in the above literature (Shin et al. 2010; Karakülah et al. 2014; Gillies et al. 2016; Somashekhar et al. 2017; You et al. 2018). AI can use complex algorithms to read features from massive amounts of healthcare data and then use the results to improve clinical practice. It can also be outfitted with self-learning and correcting capabilities to increase its precision in response to input.

1.3. Evolution of AI

Computers are machines that operate based on the input they receive. They are unable to think by themselves or use reasoning. Computers operate entirely on the information given by humans. However, there has been a persistent push in the recent age to instill human intelligence into computers and make them think. This gave rise to the artificial intelligence (AI) field. Machine learning is the foundation of our project. But first, let us take a look at AI. AI is a catch-all phrase for any software program that allows a machine to think like a person. AI is any software that causes the computer to learn from the data presented or update itself with its numerous inputs in the same way that people do. AI is a broad phrase that encompasses several topics, including ML, neural networks and deep learning. Alexa and Siri are two current and immediately relevant instances of AI. The first artificial neurons, developed by McCulloch and Pitts in 1943, marked the beginning of AI (French et al. 1973). Donald Hebb (Munakata and Pfaffly 2004) first presented Hebbian learning in 1949. This notion is about the strength of the connections between neurons. In 1955, two men named Allen Newell and Herbert A. Simon created the first AI software, "Logic Theorist," which proved 38 of 52 mathematical programs supplied to it. John McCarthy developed the term artificial intelligence at the Dartmouth Conference in 1956. McCarthy is also recognized as the "Father of Artificial Intelligence". AI made a great jump in the beginning, but a few years of AI winter followed. Winter in this context refers to a period when scientists working on AI faced a massive backlog of work owing to a lack of funding. When world chess champion Gary Kasparov lost a chess championship to IBM Deep Blue in 1997, the golden age of AI began (Newborn 2000). In 2002, the "ROOMBA", an AI-enabled vacuum cleaner, was released for home usage (Jones 2006). By 2006, AI had become a key aspect of Facebook, Twitter and Netflix. More examples include IBM Watson (Strickland 2019), the Android app Google Now (Zhong et al. 2014) and others. Python, Tensor Flow, Java and C are examples of AI programming languages.

1.3.1. *Advantages and disadvantages*

1.3.1.1. *Advantages*

1) With the assistance of AI, the likelihood of human mistakes is greatly reduced.

2) AI is a far greater risk taker when it comes to experiments or expeditions where human life could be jeopardized, such as defusing a bomb, carrying out any space voyage or experiment, etc.

3) AI can do repetitive tasks such as sending reminder emails, thank you emails, verifying documents and classifying emails as spam or starred. In a word, it can perform any unusual work that humans may lose interest in.

4) AI can work indefinitely without taking breaks or vacations, unlike humans.

5) AI allows certain commonplace apps, such as OK GOOGLE, SIRI and CORTANA, to mention a few.

6) AI makes decisions at a far faster rate than humans.

7) With the aid of AI, the medical industry has evolved considerably, since it is now feasible to diagnose and cure life-threatening disorders.

1.3.1.2. *Disadvantages*

1) The assistance of AI in healthcare systems reduces the human factor, which is a key part of the healthcare sector, especially in medical surgery.

2) Because AI works better and more quickly than humans, it has increased unemployment.

3) AI has turned out to be rather expensive since constant advances necessitate changes in hardware and circuits. Frequent changes entitle us to a large sum of money.

4) Machines, unlike humans, cannot think for themselves and are completely reliant on the data given.

5) AI-enabled household appliances are causing humans to become drowsy and reliant on them.

1.3.2. *Components of AI*

AI is a broad word that encompasses several sub-disciplines such as ML, NN and DL. Figure 1.1 simplifies the above statement.

1.3.2.1. *Machine learning*

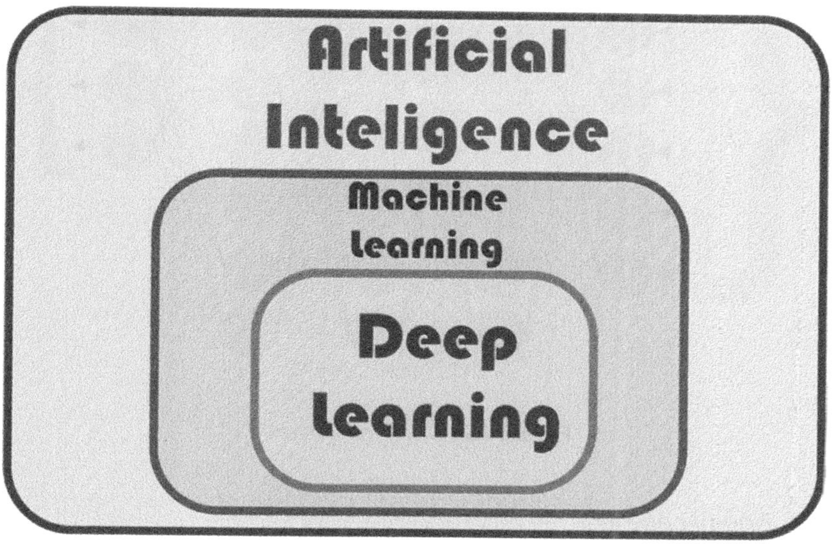

Figure 1.1. *AI–ML–DL*

Machine learning is a branch of AI that can function even when the computer has not been explicitly trained to do so. Computers in this field of AI can operate and learn on their own. They are capable of dealing with the problem, figuring it out and clarifying the data to solve it. The algorithms are so clever that they can predict the consequences. The primary distinction between AI and ML is that, unlike AI, ML can evolve. Nowadays, machine learning is widely used in optical communication. Several research projects are being carried out using a combination of machine learning and optical communication. Some prominent efforts include chromatic dispersion reduction (Wang et al. 2015; Ranzini et al. 2019), phase noise correction (Wang et al. 2016) and nonlinearity mitigation (Wang et al. 2016).

1.3.2.2. *Deep learning*

Deep learning is a subset of machine learning, which incorporates different layers to gather information from data (Deng and Yu 2014). A typical DNN structure is shown in Figure 1.2.

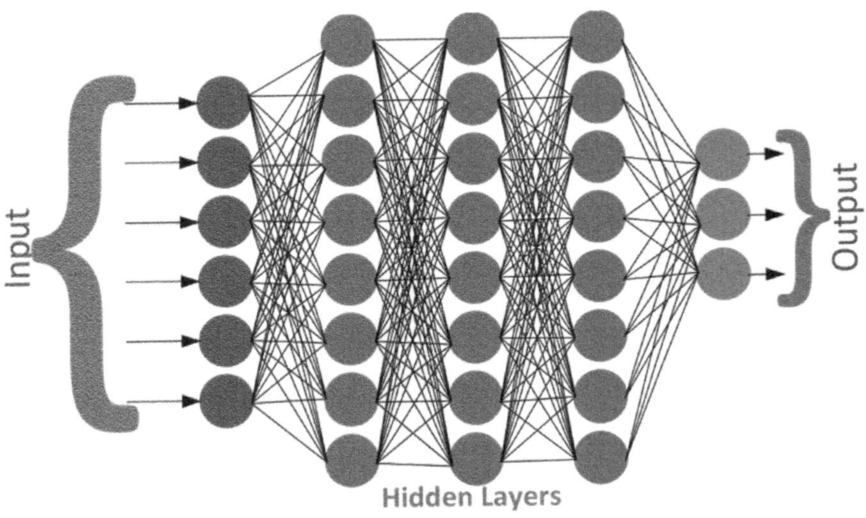

Figure 1.2. *DNN architecture*

1.3.2.3. *Neural network*

A neural network is a type of AI that attempts to interpret data in the same manner that the human brain does. Long before computers, people experienced neural networks (Maren 1990). Neural networks have made significant advances in pattern detection in voice, sonar, radar and other domains. They are also used to reduce noise and numerous nonlinearities. Neural networks can be broken into three sections for easier comprehension. In both particular and non-specific systems, there are an element processing layer, element processing columns and neural tissue (Maren 1990). Many low-cost neural network VLSI chips are now widely available (Maren et al. 2014). A key use of neural networks is robust pattern detection (Maren et al. 2014).

1.4. Machine learning

In today's technological environment, machine learning has evolved as an interdisciplinary tool. It was deliberately used in this project effort because of its incredible capacity to detect and reduce nonlinearity. In this section, we will go through the various components of machine learning. We used the supervised learning approach in our project. Machine learning has exploded in the world of telecommunications in recent years. It plays a significant role in our daily life. It has become an essential component of today's current research. ML algorithms have aided AI in expanding beyond the programming that it is fed.

1.4.1. *Categories of ML*

ML develops itself via training. ML is currently trained in three fundamental ways: "supervised learning," "unsupervised learning" and "reinforcement learning". We need to understand the various types of data that they use. ML uses two types of data: labeled data and unlabeled data. Labeled data is data that includes both the input and output in a readable manner. However, labeling the data is a time-consuming and labor-intensive task. Unlabeled data, on the other hand, has no labeling and requires no human intervention, but the complexity grows.

1.4.2. *Supervised learning*

Supervised learning is one of the popular types of ML. The term "supervised" refers to any type of control or guiding. The data used in this case is labeled data that is closely supervised by the relevant output so that changes in the output can be identified. When the ML algorithm uses the same set of data with the same properties, this is referred to as supervised learning (Kotsiantis et al. 2007). In supervised learning, the algorithm is given a tiny data sheet comparable to the original one to train itself on. The program then attempts to determine a relationship between all of the data presented. It attempts to discover the relationship between the data using the cause-and-effect approach. As a result, the algorithm can continue to learn new things as it grows. It is further subdivided into two sections: regression and classification.

1.4.2.1. *Regression*

It maintains learning from the data sheet supplied and, as a result, provides consistent output for fresh data that is fed to the algorithm. It establishes a link between the dependent and independent variables. It anticipates actual values such as temperature, money, height and price. It is used to forecast weather, the stock market and other events.

1.4.2.2. *Classification*

The method receives data as input and uses it to categorize the output in supervised learning. When the input is in the form of categories, it is used to predict the output. A classification model predicts the outcome as labels such as happy or sad, pass or fail, and so on. Classification is regarded as a very successful data mining approach for separating different types of data (Saritas and Yasar 2019). The following are the most significant algorithms used in supervised learning:

1) linear regression;

2) logistic regression;

3) SVM;

4) naive Bayes;

5) decision trees;

6) KNN.

1.4.2.3. *Linear regression*

Linear regression applies to continuous variables. It is used to solve linear regression issues. A straight line is used to illustrate the linear relationship between the dependent and independent variables. This type of graph is known as a scatter plot (Montgomery et al. 2021). The purpose of ML is to calibrate this connection.

1.4.2.4. *Logistic regression*

Logistic regression is used to analyze categorical variables (Gasso 2019). It resolves categorization issues. It is a better alternative than linear regression since the curved curve or s-curve includes all points. All of the forecasts are discrete values. It is most effective for binary categorization. Whether yes or no, the outcome is probabilistic.

1.4.2.5. *SVM*

SVM can be used for both classification and regression; however, it is more commonly used for classification. It is a large data multi-sphere application (Suthaharan 2016).

1.4.2.6. *Native Bayes*

The theorem of naive Bayes is used in practice to discover probabilistic output. It is a very essential and commonly used algorithm in data mining (Chen et al. 2020). With the assistance of an example, we can comprehend it. Assume that we are flipping a coin. The likelihood of the outcome being heads or tails is exactly 50–50. The following example will help to clarify the issue. Assume that two occurrences, A and B, are taking place. Event A is a power outage on a July day. Event B is hoping for a cool reprieve from the sun and the arrival of an ice cream cart. As a result, the likelihood of event B occurring is entirely reliant on event A. If event A happens, eventually event B will follow.

1.4.2.7. *Decision tree*

Although the decision tree technique can be used for both regression and classification, it is more commonly used for classification (Su and Zhang 2006). It is similar to a tree in that the interior nodes represent dataset characteristics, the branches represent decision rules and the leaf node represents the output. It is called a tree because its structure is similar to that of a tree, beginning with the base and progressing to the stem and branches with leaves. A tree is constructed using the "CART" algorithm, which stands for classification and regression tree algorithm.

1.4.2.8. *KNN*

The simplest, practically error-free and most extensively used supervised learning technique is K-nearest neighbor (KNN), which is mostly used for classification issues (Kuang and Zhao 2009). This algorithm learns slowly since it keeps all of the data from the data sheet and only uses it when categorizing fresh data. The steps are discussed below:

1) It obtains the labeled data.

2) It specifies the K-nearest neighbor or k sample points (Kuang and Zhao 2009).

3) QI inquiry points are a new member with an unknown category (Kuang and Zhao 2009).

4) Each point is denoted by the formula p1 = p2p3.... pn (Kuang and Zhao 2009).

5) The distance between the nearest neighbors is computed.

6) The distance is computed using either the Euclidean or Manhattan distances (Kuang and Zhao 2009).

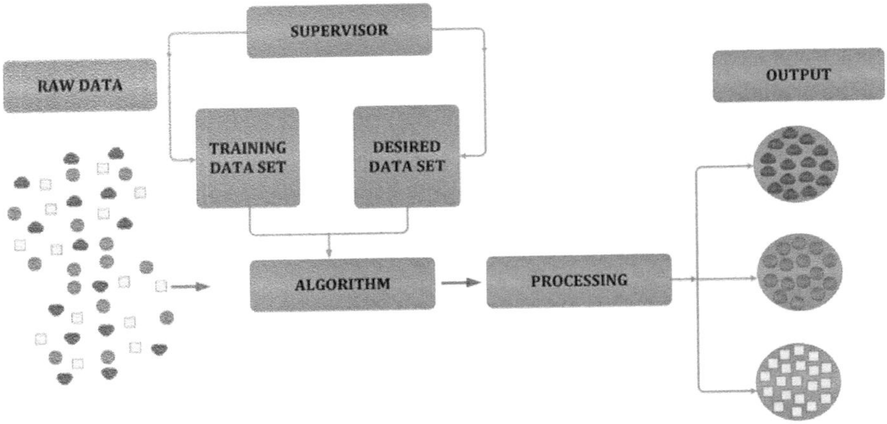

Figure 1.3. *Supervised learning*

1.4.2.9. *Applications of supervised learning*

1) Bioinformatics is the best application of supervised learning. It comprises fingerprints, iris texture and earlobes, among other things. Smartphones currently use iris recognition, facial recognition and fingerprints as passwords.

2) Speech recognition is another use, in which our speech is used as input to an algorithm that can recognize us. In this sense, Google Assistant and SIRI are the greatest examples.

3) Spam detection is another useful application, in which the algorithm recognizes spam emails and marks them as spam.

4) Vision object identification is another application in which specific items can be detected. In this context, Raspberry Pi algorithms are used.

1.4.2.10. *Drawbacks of supervised learning*

1) The algorithms should be trained on real-world data.

2) It takes a long time to process the data.

3) If unauthentic data is given, the accuracy suffers.

4) Data pre-estimation is difficult.

1.4.3. *Unsupervised learning*

As a training set for unsupervised learning, unlabeled data is used. As a result, it is machine-readable and does not require human involvement. This makes it ideal for large data sheets. Because no human intervention is necessary, it functions by developing some hidden patterns. Because they are unlabeled, they can be readily included in any dataset by simply modifying the concealed pattern. In comparison to supervised learning, they can tackle more complicated tasks. The algorithm receives input in unsupervised learning, but the output is neither predetermined nor is it rewarded for accurate judgment or output (Ghahramani 2003). It cannot be applied immediately to any situation since it has no preset output. Assume that the algorithm is given some photographs of boys and girls, but has no foreknowledge on how to discriminate between them. With no preexisting dataset, it will then cluster the photos into groups based on characteristics. It is further divided into two parts: clustering and association.

1.4.3.1. *Clustering*

Clustering is a significant unsupervised learning approach. It is the technique of detecting a hidden pattern in unclassified raw data. These algorithms refine the data and, if necessary, construct clusters or groups from it. The produced clusters are of good quality, with extensive intra-class analogy and shallow inter-class analogy (Mann and Kaur 2013).

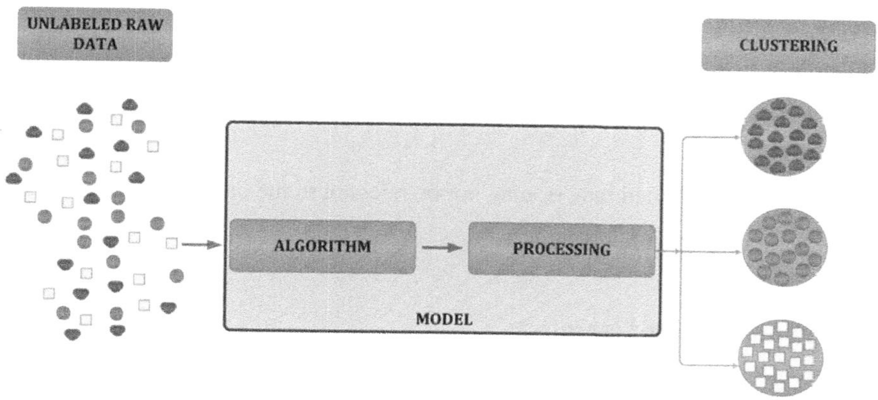

Figure 1.4. *Unsupervised learning*

1.4.3.2. *Association*

Association learning algorithms discover relationships between things in a huge data collection. The interdependence of data is determined in this scenario, and mapping is performed accordingly. Market basket analysis is one such association method used by large retailers to discover associations between the store's various items. If a client purchases baby food, they are more likely to purchase baby creams, lotions and diapers.

A few unsupervised learning approaches are mentioned below:

1) K-means clustering;

2) hierarchical clustering;

3) principal component analysis.

1.4.3.3. *Applications of unsupervised learning*

1) It is used to find patterns in a data collection.

2) Several problems have been identified that could not have been identified at an earlier time.

3) Mapping can be accomplished via unsupervised learning by examining the interdependence of the data presented.

4) It can remove undesired data from the data collection.

5) Amazon uses unsupervised learning to determine the relationship between the many things in its marketplace.

1.4.3.4. *Drawbacks of supervised learning*

1) Unlabeled data makes it hard to locate the data sorting process.

2) Because human intervention is not necessary, the possibility of inaccuracy is considerable.

3) The result obtained may or may not be relevant to the output sought.

4) Calculation is quite difficult.

1.4.4. *Reinforcement learning*

The most intriguing of all learning approaches is reinforcement learning. It involves learning the job and determining how to gain the most rewards. It is essentially a trial and error strategy in which the algorithm learns on its own by trying several methods and determining which way gives it the most rewards (Mann and Kaur 2013). Reinforcement learning differs from supervised learning in that it always works with new and fresh data, whereas supervised learning is given tagged data.

A few reinforcement learning approaches are mentioned below:

1) Monte Carlo;

2) Q-learning;

3) deep Q network.

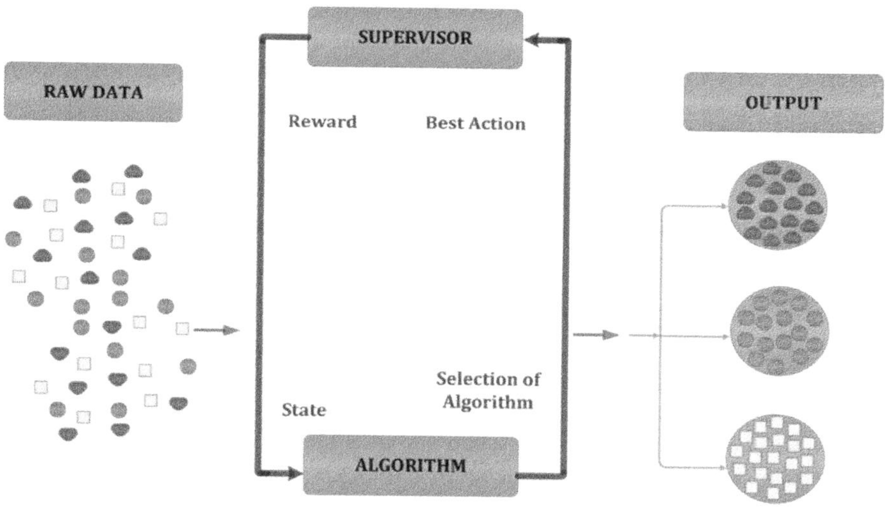

Figure 1.5. *Reinforced learning*

1.4.4.1. *Applications of unsupervised learning*

1) When it comes to robotics, it is a good option.

2) It is used to make commercial decisions.

3) It aids in the creation of customized student study materials and study method ideas.

4) It aids with air traffic control.

5) It is also an excellent choice for game development.

1.4.4.2. *Drawbacks of supervised learning*

1) It cannot be used to solve simple issues.

2) A large amount of data is required, and the computing time is too long.

3) It is heavily reliant on the Markovian model, which is a problem.

1.5. Application of ML

Machine learning is the jargon in today's modern technological environment. It has been expanding by leaps and bounds during the last few decades. Through machine learning, a computer can mimic human behavior and discover and solve problems. Machine learning has grown into an interdisciplinary tool that is extensively used in all fields. Medical applications, military applications, social networking, e-commerce and telecommunications (Sinha et al. 2021; Ghosh 2022; Ghosh et al. 2023; Jichkar et al. 2023) are just a few examples. There are several applications to be discussed in the medical profession. ML can be used to determine the blood group of Danish jersey cattle (Kukar 1995). It is commonly used to forecast the progression of symptoms associated with femoral neck fracture recovery (Kukar et al. 1996). It has ushered in a new era by diagnosing dangerous ischemic heart disease (Kukar et al. 1999). ML has also been used to identify structural progressors in knee osteoarthritis (Perone 2022).

The Covid-19 pandemic has wreaked havoc on the whole planet over the last two years. ML has been used to detect and predict Covid-19 instances (Perone 2022). ML has also been deemed a useful technique in epigenetics, which is the study of the effects of the environment on genetics (Holder et al. 2017). After considering machine learning's vivid use in the medical field, we can move on to its significance in defense. Machine learning has made an impression in military applications. Some of them are covered in this section. Defense is concerned with a country's overall security. When it comes to discovering an invader, defense professionals leave no stone unturned. Machine learning has greatly aided in the detection and capture of intruders through the use of facial recognition (Goel et al. 2019). The United States of America uses machine learning in its special forces to predict the likelihood of musculoskeletal injury during training (Connaboy et al. 2019).

Moving on to additional applications of machine learning, it has been proven to be useful with environmental challenges. Machine learning can be used to check for knowledge of water erosion in soil (Mosavi et al. 2020). It can also be used to assess the crucial issue of global warming (Zheng 2018). In addition, machine learning can identify flood situations quite efficiently (Felix and Sasipraba 2019). Agriculture is responsible for a very vital component of daily life: food. We rely entirely on agriculture and cattle for our daily sustenance, although livestock does perish from climate fluctuations and disease. Machine learning has aided in the general care of crops, the kind of soil for agriculture, the amount of water required for crop development and the care of farm animals (Liakos et al. 2018). Machine learning benefits agriculture even more since it can accurately estimate the harvest and fix the right quantity of nitrogen in the soil (Chlingaryan et al. 2018).

After we have covered all of these applications, let us look at some of the most recent and popular uses of machine learning. Social media is the most popular application. Teenagers are especially drawn to it and can become so absorbed in it that it affects their mental health. Trolling or hateful remarks on social media are issues that can severely harm young minds. Machine learning can assist in spotting inappropriate comments and preventing cyberbullying (Chavan and Shylaja 2015). Another major task performed by machine learning is the detection of fraud in e-transactions, which has become a problem in the online world (Nanduri et al. 2020). Our lifestyle is growing more frantic as we get more contemporary. Some consumers prefer online shopping rather than visiting malls. Such clients may find it difficult to get the most appropriate items to meet their needs. Machine learning is also useful in presenting the most relevant alternatives for the client to choose from (Yang et al. 2004).

After discussing all of these fascinating uses of machine learning, let us return to our core issue of communication. Communication is classified into two types: wireless communication and wired communication. Let us now look at how machine learning is being used in these two domains. Edge learning is a very interesting concept that has recently evolved, which involves attaching devices to gather data based on AI from them and analyzing that data (Xu et al. 2020). For the new edge learning, wireless communication could be given an entirely new layout (Zhu et al. 2020). Machine learning can also be used to comprehend potential aspects beyond 5G (B5G) (Morocho-Cayamcela et al. 2019). Wireless sensor networks (WSN) are a new concept in the realm of wireless networks that can help predict natural disasters such as storms, heavy rain and flooding. Forest fires can be predicted using WSN and machine learning (Kansal et al. 2015). Machine learning can be used to select the best antenna for wireless communication (Kansal et al. 2015). Following wireless communication, we will look at how machine learning can be applied in wired communication. Optical communication is indicated when the term wired communication is used. Machine learning can be used to evaluate both linear and nonlinear noises in optical networks (Joung 2016). Non-Gaussian nonlinearities in optical fiber can also be reduced using machine learning (Savory and Caballero 2018). In optical communication, distortion is a major issue. Machine learning can be used to reduce distortions in PAM 4 and PAM 8 signals (Amari et al. 2019). These are some examples of machine learning applications in many disciplines.

1.6. Application of AI in healthcare

The healthcare sector is beginning to recognize the significance of AI solutions in future medical technologies. It is believed that it can improve the existing structure of healthcare.

1.6.1. *Digital health*

Healthcare applications collect and analyze patient-supplied information such as food consumption, psychological response and patient condition surveillance data via smart bands, sensors, etc. A few of these applications are classified as precision medicine because they use ML algorithms to detect patterns in data, predict them and provide personalized care suggestions.

1.6.2. *Genetic solutions*

ML algorithms are used with genetic data to detect connections and predict therapy responses for the individual patient. Other indicators, such as protein level and metabolic activity, are used in conjunction with ML to provide tailored therapy (Chen et al. 2017).

1.6.3. *Bio-medical visualization*

It can be difficult to interpret data that comes in the form of a picture or a video. Specialists in the area must practice for several years to be able to distinguish medical occurrences, and they must also consistently acquire new content when new knowledge and analysis become available. However, the market is expanding, so there is a severe scarcity of expertise in the industry. As a result, a new method is required, and AI appears to be the instrument that will be used to cope with this situation.

1.6.3.1. *Computer vision (CV) in disease detection*

CV has traditionally been based on statistical signal processing, but it is increasingly changing towards the use of ANN as the preferred learning approach. In this case, DL is used to create CV algorithms to identify medical photos. One useful aspect of AI and CV in the surgical field is to improve specific surgical characteristics and talents such as suturing, drilling, etc. Malaria detection using CV is depicted in Figure 1.6.

1.6.3.2. *Augmented reality in healthcare*

Augmented virtual reality (AVR) can be used at every level of the healthcare system. These methods can be adopted from the beginning of medical school, for those preparing for a specialized specialization and for seasoned surgeons.

This is demonstrated by the example shown in Figure 1.6.

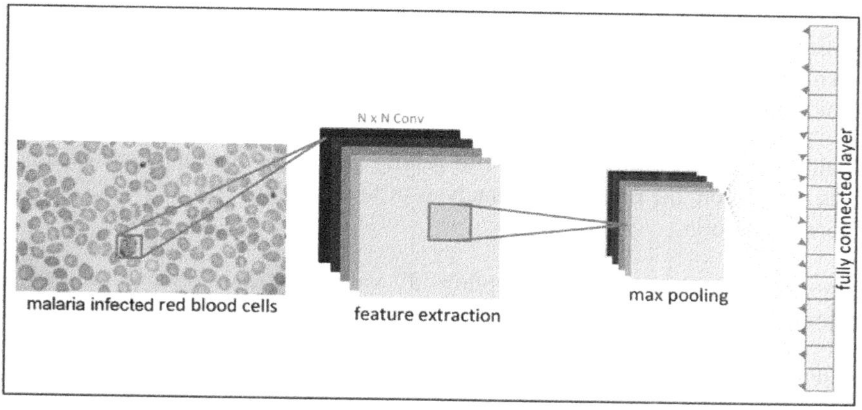

Figure 1.6. *Malaria detection using CV*

1.6.3.3. *Mental state prediction using AI*

SL. No.	Mental state	Training set	Testing set
1	Fear	400	100
2	Happy	100	100
3	Sad	400	100
4	Surprise	400	100
5	Anger	400	100

Table 1.1. *Training and testing dataset split*

The data used here is generated in controlled conditions. Each person undergoes various mental states. The eye pupil dilation images are captured in each case. The emotions incorporated here are fear, happiness, sadness, surprise and anger. Then,

70% data was used for training and 30% data was used for validation purposes. Table 1.1 shows that in all cases 500 different human eye pupil images have been taken in different mantle conditions. Among those 500 images, 400 have been used to train the AI model and 100 have been used to test the model.

Table 1.1 shows the train–test split.

This is a convolution neural network designed with a deep neural network classifier from TensorFlow in Python language. Table 1.2 shows 2,000 images divided into five different classes. The activation function used in this network is sigmoid, and the training process has been done over 100 epochs.

Table 1.2 shows all the training and testing model performances of the model. This is nothing but the performance analysis of the machine learning model to detect the correct emotion.

As shown in Figure 1.7, "inceptionV3" validation and training accuracy is stagnant at 100% and the loss curve is also at near the zero line.

Table 1.2 shows the performance table.

Epochs	Loss (train)	Accuracy (train)	Loss (valid)	Accuracy (valid)
10	0.3584	0.898	1556.9858	0.2
20	0.3641	0.898	128.546	0.184
30	0.06	0.974	0.541	0.916
40	0.0028	1	0.0164	0.992
50	0.0012	1	0.0119	0.996
60	0.0216	0.992	0.0123	0.992
70	0.0269	0.994	0.0964	0.97
80	0.1172	0.97	10.4817	0.436
90	0.0149	0.994	0.1034	0.962
100	0.008	0.998	0.0062	0.998

Table 1.2. *Performance analysis*

1.7. Conclusion

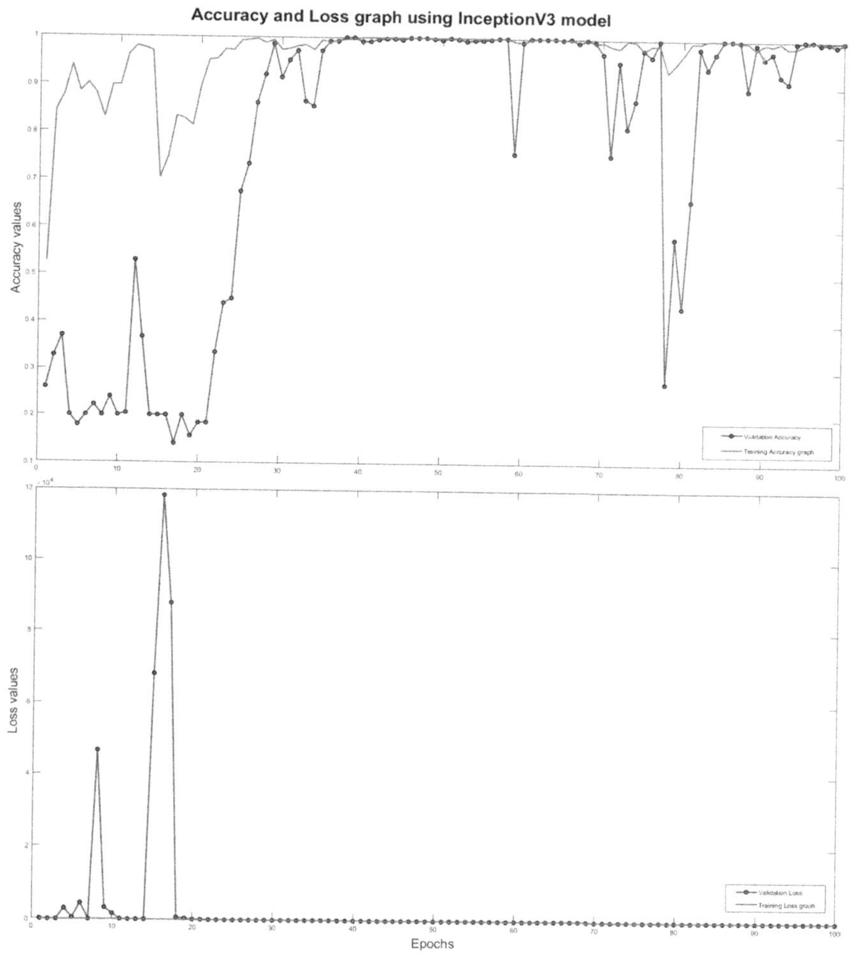

Figure 1.7. *Performance graph*

ML and AI are influencing almost every area of contemporary civilization, including amusement, business and healthcare. All of this information can be used to create very comprehensive personal profiles, which can be useful not only for behavioral learning and monitoring, but also for anticipating medical patterns. There is a lot of hope that the use of AI will result in significant advancements in all aspects of healthcare, from diagnosis to therapy.

1.8. References

Amari, A., Lin, X., Dobre, O.A., Venkatesan, R., Alvarado, A. (2019). A machine learning-based detection technique for optical fiber nonlinearity mitigation. *IEEE Photonics Technology Letters*, 31(8), 627–630.

Chavan, V.S. and Shylaja, S.S. (2015). Machine learning approach for detection of cyber-aggressive comments by peers on social media network. *2015 International Conference on Advances in Computing, Communications and Informatics (ICACCI)*, 2354–2358. IEEE.

Chen, S., Dong, X., Peng, Z., Zhang, W., Meng, G. (2017). Nonlinear chirp mode decomposition: A variational method. *IEEE Transactions on Signal Processing*, 65(22), 6024–6037.

Chen, S., Webb, G.I., Liu, L., Ma, X. (2020). A novel selective naïve Bayes algorithm. *Knowledge-Based Systems*, 192, 105361.

Chlingaryan, A., Sukkarieh, S., Whelan, B. (2018). Machine learning approaches for crop yield prediction and nitrogen status estimation in precision agriculture: A review. *Computers and Electronics in Agriculture*, 151, 61–69.

Connaboy, C., Eagle, S.R., Johnson, C., Flanagan, S., Mi, Q.I., Nindl, B.C. (2019). Using machine learning to predict lower extremity injury in US Special Forces. *Medicine and Science in Sports and Exercise*, 51(5), 1073–1079.

Deng, L. and Yu, D. (2014). Deep learning: Methods and applications. *Foundations and Trends in Signal Processing*, 7(3–4), 197–387.

Felix, A.Y. and Sasipraba, T. (2019). Flood detection using gradient boost machine learning approach. *2019 International Conference on Computational Intelligence and Knowledge Economy (ICCIKE)*, 779–783. IEEE.

French, W.G., Pearson, A.D., Tasker, G.W., Mac-Chesney, J.B. (1973). Low-loss fused silica optical waveguide with borosilicate cladding. *Applied Physics Letters*, 23(6), 338–339.

Gasso, G. (2021). Logistic regression. Presentation, ITI Department, Laboratory LITIS, INSA Rouen [Online]. Available at: https://moodle.insa-rouen.fr/pluginfile.php/7984/mod_resource/content/6/Parties_1_et_3_DM/RegLog_Eng.pdf [Accessed 8 December 2023].

Ghahramani, Z. (2003). Unsupervised learning. In *Summer School on Machine Learning*, Bousquet, O., von Luxburg, U., Rätsch, G. (eds). Springer, Berlin, 71–112.

Ghosh, M. (2022). Comparative DNN model analysis for detection of various types of optical noise. *TechRxiv*. doi: 10.36227/techrxiv.19160615.v1.

Ghosh, M., Raut, M., Parteki, R., Das, D., Thakare, L.P., Jichkar, R., Rathore, S.S., Bawankar, S. (2023). An analysis of deep-neural-network model for the determination of the bit-rate of optical fiber signals. *2023 11th International Conference on Emerging Trends in Engineering & Technology-Signal and Information Processing (ICETET-SIP)*, 1–4. IEEE.

Gillies, R.J., Kinahan, P.E., Hricak, H. (2016). Radiomics: Images are more than pictures, they are data. *Radiology*, 278(2), 563.

Goel, V., Raj, H., Muthigi, K., Kumar, S.S., Prasad, D., Nath, V. (2019). Development of human detection system for security and military applications. In *Proceedings of the Third International Conference on Microelectronics, Computing and Communication Systems*, 195–200. Springer.

Holder, L.B., Haque, M.M., Skinner, M.K. (2017). Machine learning for epigenetics and future medical applications. *Epigenetics*, 12(7), 505–514.

Jichkar, R., Paraskar, S., Parteki, R., Ghosh, M., Deotale, T., Pathan, A.S., Bawankar, S., Thakare, L.P. (2023). 5g: An emerging technology and its advancement. *2023 11th International Conference on Emerging Trends in Engineering & Technology-Signal and Information Processing (ICETET-SIP)*, 1–6. IEEE.

Jones, J.L. (2006). Robots at the tipping point: The road to iRobot Roomba. *IEEE Robotics & Automation Magazine*, 13(1), 76–78.

Joung, J. (2016). Machine learning-based antenna selection in wireless communications. *IEEE Communications Letters*, 20(11), 2241–2244.

Kansal, A., Singh, Y., Kumar, N., Mohindru, V. (2015). Detection of forest fires using machine learning technique: A perspective. *2015 Third International Conference on Image Information Processing (ICIIP)*, 241–245. IEEE.

Karakülah, G., Dicle, O., Koşaner, O., Suner, A., Can Birant, Ç., Berber, T., Canbek, S. (2014). Computer based extraction of phenoptypic features of human congenital anomalies from the digital literature with natural language processing techniques. *e-Health–For Continuity of Care*, 570–574. IOS Press.

Kotsiantis, S.B., Zaharakis, I., Pintelas, P. (2007). Supervised machine learning: A review of classification techniques. *Emerging Artificial Intelligence Applications in Computer Engineering*, 160(1), 3–24.

Kuang, Q. and Zhao, L. (2009). A practical GPU based KNN algorithm. *Proceedings of the 2009 International Symposium on Computer Science and Computational Technology (ISCSCI 2009)*, 151. Citeseer.

Kukar, M. (1995). Machine learning in blood group determination of Danish Jersey cattle. *Citeseer*.

Kukar, M., Kononenko, I., Silvester, T. (1996). Machine learning in prognosis of the femoral neck fracture recovery. *Artificial Intelligence in Medicine*, 8(5), 431–451.

Kukar, M., Kononenko, I., Grošelj, C., Kralj, K., Fettich, J. (1999). Analysing and improving the diagnosis of ischaemic heart disease with machine learning. *Artificial Intelligence in Medicine*, 16(1), 25–50.

Liakos, K.G., Busato, P., Moshou, D., Pearson, S., Bochtis, D. (2018). Machine learning in agriculture: A review. *Sensors*, 18(8), 2674.

Love-Koh, J., Peel, A., Parrilla, J.C.R., Ennis, K., Lovett, R., Manca, A., Chalkidou, A., Wood, H., Taylor, M. (2018). The future of precision medicine: Potential impacts for health technology assessment. *Pharmacoeconomics*, 36(12), 1439–1451.

Mann, A.K. and Kaur, N. (2013). Review paper on clustering techniques. *Global Journal of Computer Science and Technology Software & Data Engineering*, 13(5), 42–47.

Maren, A.J. (1990). Introduction to neural networks. In *Handbook of Neural Computing Applications*, Maren, A.J., Harston, C.T., Pap, R.M. (eds). Academic Press, San Diego, 1–12.

Maren, A.J., Harston, C.T., Pap, R.M. (2014). *Handbook of Neural Computing Applications*. Academic Press, San Diego.

Montgomery, D.C., Peck, E.A., Vining, G.G. (2021). *Introduction to Linear Regression Analysis*. John Wiley & Sons, Hoboken.

Morocho-Cayamcela, M.E., Lee, H., Lim, W. (2019). Machine learning for 5g/b5g mobile and wireless communications: Potential, limitations, and future directions. *IEEE Access*, 7, 137184–137206.

Mosavi, A., Sajedi-Hosseini, F., Choubin, B., Taromideh, F., Rahi, G., Dineva, A.A. (2020). Susceptibility mapping of soil water erosion using machine learning models. *Water*, 12(7), 1995.

Munakata, Y. and Pfaffly, J. (2004). Hebbian learning and development. *Developmental Science*, 7(2), 141–148.

Nanduri, J., Jia, Y., Oka, A., Beaver, J., Liu, Y.-W. (2020). Microsoft uses machine learning and optimization to reduce e-commerce fraud. *INFORMS Journal on Applied Analytics*, 50(1), 64–79.

Newborn, M. (2000). Deep Blue's contribution to AI. *Annals of Mathematics and Artificial Intelligence*, 28(1), 27–30.

Perone, G. (2022). Using the SARIMA model to forecast the fourth global wave of cumulative deaths from COVID-19: Evidence from 12 hard-hit big countries. *Econometrics*, 10(2), 18.

Ranzini, S.M., Da Ros, F., Bülow, H., Zibar, D. (2019). Tunable optoelectronic chromatic dispersion compensation based on machine learning for short-reach transmission. *Applied Sciences*, 9(20), 4332.

Saritas, M.M. and Yasar, A. (2019). Performance analysis of ANN and naive Bayes classification algorithm for data classification. *International Journal of Intelligent Systems and Applications in Engineering*, 7(2), 88–91.

Savory, S.J. and Caballero, F.J.V. (2018). Machine learning based noise estimation in optical fiber communication networks. *2018 IEEE Photonics Society Summer Topical Meeting Series (SUM)*, 57–58. IEEE.

Shin, H., Kim, K.H., Song, C., Lee, I., Lee, K., Kang, J., Kang, Y.K. (2010). Electrodiagnosis support system for localizing neural injury in an upper limb. *Journal of the American Medical Informatics Association*, 17(3), 345–347.

Sinha, N., Ghosh, M., Majumder, S., Bhowmik, B.B. (2021). Deep learning based noise identification in the optical fiber communication using variational mode decomposition. *2021 IEEE 2nd International Conference on Applied Electromagnetics, Signal Processing, & Communication (AESPC)*, 1–5. IEEE.

Somashekhar, S.P., Kumarc, R., Rauthan, A., Arun, K.R., Patil, P., Ramya, Y.E. (2017). Abstract S6-07: Double blinded validation study to assess performance of IBM artificial intelligence platform, Watson for oncology in comparison with Manipal multidisciplinary tumour board – First study of 638 breast cancer cases. *Cancer Research*, 77(4 Supplement), S6–07.

Strickland, E. (2019). IBM Watson, heal thyself: How IBM overpromised and underdelivered on AI health care. *IEEE Spectrum*, 56(4), 24–31.

Su, J. and Zhang, H. (2006). A fast decision tree learning algorithm. *AAAI*, 6, 500–505.

Suthaharan, S. (2016). Machine learning models and algorithms for big data classification. *Integrated Series in Information Systems*, 36, 1–12.

Wang, D., Zhang, M., Li, Z., Cui, Y., Liu, J., Yang, Y., Wang, H. (2015). Nonlinear decision boundary created by a machine learning-based classifier to mitigate nonlinear phase noise. *2015 European Conference on Optical Communication (ECOC)*, 1–3. IEEE.

Wang, D., Zhang, M., Cai, Z., Cui, Y., Li, Z., Han, H., Fu, M., Luo, B. (2016). Combatting nonlinear phase noise in coherent optical systems with an optimized decision processor based on machine learning. *Optics Communications*, 369, 199–208.

Xu, D., Li, T., Li, Y., Su, X., Tarkoma, S., Jiang, T., Crowcroft, J., Hui, P. (2020). Edge intelligence: Architectures, challenges, and applications. arXiv preprint arXiv:2003.12172.

Yang, H.-W., Pan, Z.-G., Wang, X.-Z., Xu, B. (2004). A personalized products selection assistance based on e-commerce machine learning. *Proceedings of 2004 International Conference on Machine Learning and Cybernetics (IEEE Cat. No 04EX826)*, 4, 2629–2633. IEEE.

You, X., Zhao, Y., Sui, J., Shi, X., Sun, Y., Xu, J., Liang, G., Xu, Q., Yao, Y. (2018). Integrated analysis of long non-coding RNA interactions reveals the potential role in progression of human papillary thyroid cancer. *Cancer Medicine*, 7(11), 5394–5410.

Zheng, H. (2018). Analysis of global warming using machine learning. *Computational Water, Energy, and Environmental Engineering*, 7(3), 127.

Zhong, Y., Raman, T.V., Burkhardt, C., Biadsy, F., Bigham, J.P. (2014). Justspeak: Enabling universal voice control on android. *Proceedings of the 11th Web for All Conference*, 1–4.

Zhu, G., Liu, D., Du, Y., You, C., Zhang, J., Huang, K. (2020). Toward an intelligent edge: Wireless communication meets machine learning. *IEEE Communications Magazine*, 58(1), 19–25.

2

Medical Laboratory Artificial Intelligence: The Applicability in Nigerian Medical Laboratories

Artificial intelligence (AI) is defined as the study and development of computer systems that can copy intelligent human behavior. AI, together with machine or computer learning, provides opportunities to carry out many works of life in various professions – medical laboratory science being one of them. This chapter adopts a review and narrative commentary, based on published scientific articles with medical laboratory service observations performed to analyze many real-world instances in the medical laboratories; this is to infer how AI affects laboratory services and operations globally, with special interest in Nigeria. This was to enable us to recommend strategies for enhanced laboratory services and efficiency in disease diagnosis in Nigerian medical laboratories. Thus, we reviewed the relevant literature extensively to reveal AI-based technologies and their applications in medical laboratories. This chapter shows that the majority of medical laboratories in Nigeria at present do not use AI-enabled systems to support medical laboratory staff in their processes. This could be as a result of poor facilities and a less motivated medical laboratory workforce, especially in Nigeria. Although the medical laboratories in Nigeria have started using AI machines, they are encouraged to develop in such areas soon and be ready to move with the trend, especially in the medical laboratory AI-supported facilities and services.

Chapter written by Uchejeso Mark OBETA, Nkereuwem Sunday ETUKUDOH, Obiora Reginald EJINAKA and Amaechi Eze ODONO.
For a color version of all the figures in this chapter, see www.iste.co.uk/pradhan/cognitivecomputing.zip.

2.1. Introduction

AI is the simulation of human intelligence in machines (computers or robots), programmed to imitate cognitive functions the way humans relate with other human minds, like learning and problem-solving (Lee and Yoon 2021). It is a discipline in which computer technology is used to research and develop the techniques, application systems, methods and theories to simulate, expand and extend human intelligence (Liu et al. 2021). AI focuses mainly on improvising the human cognitive abilities and improving on them to perform tasking functions within a relatively shorter time frame (Gayathri et al. 2018). They include complex software systems that computers use to support and simulate human intelligence and judgment. Machine learning (ML) is an area of AI that uses algorithms to study and analyze data and then apply the knowledge to predict and make recommendations (Sisman and Basok 2020).

The difference between AI and other computer-based technologies is that AI can learn and improve with data and experience, while other technologies can execute complex tasks but cannot execute actions or reach judgments that can improve the human decisions, if not programmed specifically for such actions (Sisman and Basok 2020).

In medical practice, AI uses a set of algorithms to learn the features of a reasonable amount of medical data and helps both the medical professionals and the patients to extract and use the information (Goyal et al. 2021). AI is believed to be the most potent technology in healthcare within this digital era, supported by rapid increasing exposure to medical and health knowledge; and, to a greater extent, it improves the medical laboratory and diagnostic techniques in large scale (Gadde et al. 2020). Due to the current rapid rise in the volume of medical data readily available, it is possible to implement and use AI and ML techniques (Figure 2.1) in medical laboratory and healthcare (Gadde et al. 2020; Sisman and Basok 2020).

Medical laboratory science (MLS) is endlessly evolving and bringing creativity and new ideas/techniques to support medical decision, patient management and disease control (Greaves et al. 2019), with over 70% of decisions in healthcare depending on the service (Etukudoh et al. 2021). This has tremendous potential to transform healthcare systems and medical laboratory practice, providing better-quality healthcare to more patients and other clients (Health First Europe 2020; Etukudoh and Obeta 2021). There is no doubt that AI and Data Science are part of the innovation in MLS including automations, thereby adding to the quality improvement of services and care (Obeta et al. 2022a).

AI plays a vital role in promoting innovation and improved techniques in medical diagnostics (Gayathri et al. 2018). In MLS, the conventional methods of disease diagnosis involve manual microscopy to study the course, nature and origin of diseases analyzed by laboratory examination of body fluids, such as blood, urine, sputum and analysis of tissues. This can be time-consuming and prone to errors. By the use of AI systems and methods, such as machine vision and ML, the traditional methods can be enhanced (Gayathri et al. 2018).

In this new era of AI-supported processes, medical laboratories are moving towards more specialized roles in the management of clinical information, quality control of test results obtained outside the laboratory, advanced technology and translational medical services. AI systems, being dynamic and constantly evolving, are capable of analyzing data, learning from the generated information and making predictions and decisions (Sisman and Basok 2020).

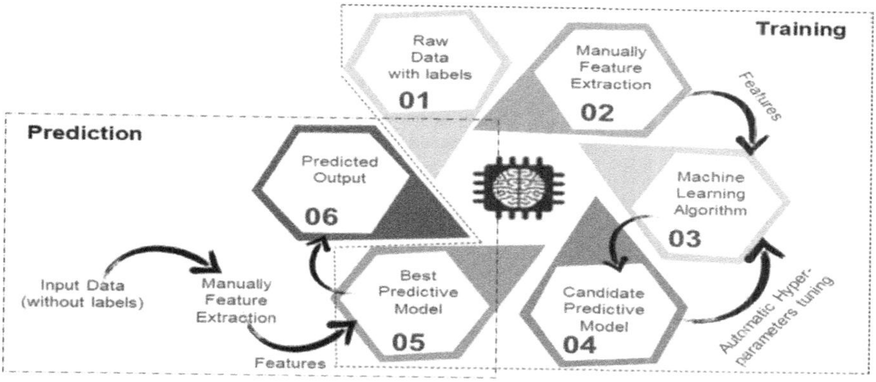

Figure 2.1. *Processes of machine learning technique as associated with artificial intelligence in medical laboratory adapted from Goyal et al. (2021)*

As with any other technological development, the increasing use of AI in different aspects of healthcare on a daily basis has triggered the fear that AI doctors (robots) could completely replace humans in the future. However, AI is meant to automate medical diagnosis and other procedures, to support and help human professionals make effective and timely decisions in patient management, rather than replace them. The technologies are built by combining human and AI and developed to assist in improving human processes (Goyal et al. 2021), of which MLS cannot be excluded. Figure 2.2 presents an AI system and work process in a medical laboratory.

The application of AI and automation in medical laboratory processes promotes timely results and makes vital patient information available for disease prediction, diagnosis and better management. The application of AI in medical laboratory practice is important in precision medicine, to individualize disease prevention, diagnosis and treatment based on genetic variability, lifestyle and environment (Goyal et al. 2021).

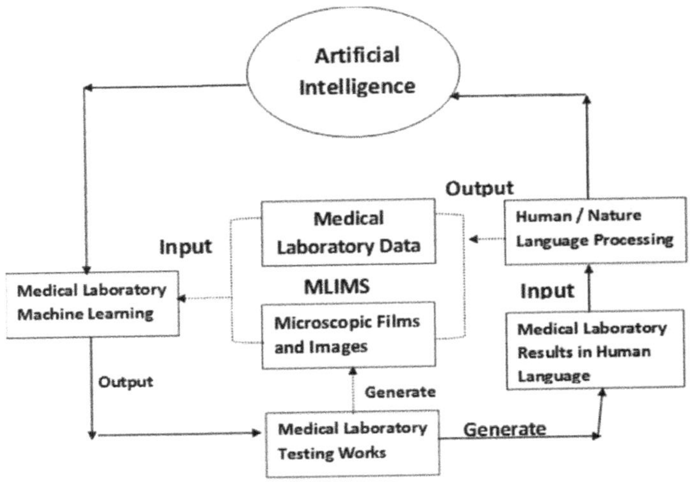

Figure 2.2. *The work process of the medical laboratory AI system*

To be effective, an AI framework should be able to have both an ML component that handles structured datasets and a natural language processing (NLP) segment to extract unstructured data. An advanced algorithmic program should be designed with healthcare/medical laboratory data that can help the medical professionals to analyze illnesses and propose treatment methods (Gayathri et al. 2018).

Expert systems (ES) stand as the most common type of AI systems used in routine medical practice. They are systems with an ability to assume expert knowledge, information and rational techniques to help human experts in their work. ES have the ability to analyze data and produce valid conclusions (Rigla et al. 2018).

Effective medical decisions on patient health conditions are based on appropriate laboratory tests. However, requesting inappropriate medical laboratory tests for patients can limit their care and increase their expenses for medical care. Islam et al. (2021) developed and validated the DNN model, a deep learning (DL)-based automated system to recommend personalized/appropriate laboratory tests for patients using simple information accessible in the EHR. This has the ability to support doctors to rapidly select appropriate tests, and potentially improves the work flow by assisting the clinicians in spending less time on test selection and more time on patient treatment.

Thus, AI has become a very important topic of discussion in the field of MLS and development of medical devices. Due to system variability, complexity, ethical and regulatory considerations, it is necessary to continually analyze and re-evaluate its performance and the applications of such devices (Badnjević et al. 2021).

This chapter examines the current status of AI-based technologies, how they are applied in medical laboratories with special interest in Nigeria and their impacts on medical evaluations (Lee et al. 2021).

2.2. Historical trend of artificial intelligence (AI)

The term artificial intelligence was first mentioned in the 1950s. From there, it evolved from the basic AI algorithms of that period to the model modification in symbolic algorithms and ES evolution in the 1970s, the unveiling of ML in the 1990s and then to DL algorithms in the 2010s (Delipetrev et al. 2020). There has been a rapid switch from heuristic approaches towards ML techniques (Rigla et al. 2018).

The period between the 1950s and 1970s served as the foundations of AI. This period saw the development of different computer programs and languages applicable in AI systems. Alan Turing made his paper titled "*Computing machinery and intelligence*" public in 1950, in which the basic question was "Can machines think?" He later proposed the "*Turing test*" to suggest that if a device could communicate in a manner that could not be differentiated from that done by humans, then it would be sensible to state that the device is intelligent. It stood as the first experiment (or test) proposed to evaluate machine intelligence (Delipetrev et al. 2020).

The initial "artificial intelligence period" started in 1955 when an American computer scientist, John McCarthy, first gave coinage to the term AI. In 1956, he organized a conference, "Dartmouth Summer Research Project on Artificial Intelligence" at Dartmouth College, New Hampshire. It was there that the name and mission of AI were discussed, and it later became an interesting scientific field. The principal conference statement was, "*Every aspect of any other feature of learning or intelligence should be accurately described so that the machine can simulate it*" (Hussein et al. 2020; Delipetrev et al. 2020).

The second period in the evolution of AI was between the 1970s and 1990s, which is called the "Symbolic AI period". The 1980s witnessed a paradigm shift of the AI to "symbolic AI" and the "expert systems" or "knowledge-based systems". The implicit view was getting human "expert knowledge" into a computer form and spreading it as a computer program to numerous computers (PCs). The two main components of the ESs were the “knowledge base” and the “inference engine”. The programming languages of the symbolic AI were Prolog and Lisp. In the 1990s, companies began to produce ESs and offered software packages known as “inference engines” and “related knowledge” services to their customers (Delipetrev et al. 2020).

The period from the 1990s to 2020s applies to ML and DL. AI in the 1990s–2010s had solved complicated problems and provided solutions useful in different application areas, such as medical diagnosis, industrial robotics, data mining, logistics and recommendation systems. Researchers in the field of AI started to create and apply more complex mathematical tools (LeCun et al. 2015). The history and use of AI in healthcare and medical laboratory services since the 1990s has been there, without a clear designation as Medical Laboratory Artificial Intelligence (MLAI). This chapter seeks to change the narrative towards formalizing MLAI.

2.3. AI in medical science/medical laboratory science in history

There has been a gradual shift from a disease-centered approach to a patient-centered model in medical care in modern times, and also from empirical to data-based information and from a paternalistic doctor–patient relationship to an egalitarian partnership (Sisman and Basok 2020). Thus, in the digital era, medical laboratories can play a vital role as a “pivot of diagnostics” by uniting the physician and patient to form a patient–physician–medical laboratory scientist triangle (Ceriotti 2019).

The practice of MLS is associated with manual work, but the AI in the history of MLS showed an improved version away from manual experience. Improved performances have been achieved in MYCIN, Internist-I, PIP, CASNET, KHT, HERMES, SETH, ISS, CBR, as well as AI systems and applications using IoMLTs and MLIMS (Hussain et al. 2017).

With AI in MLS, patients are carried along, results are easily reproduced, quality is improved, and operational efficiency and new trends are encouraged. There is no doubt that Big Data management through medical laboratory information management system is encouraged with open opportunities for interdisciplinary studies. There is also an expansion of automation, point-of-care testing (POCT) and full digitalization of medical laboratory components (Safavi and Kalis 2019).

AI techniques in medicine and MLS revolve around the following areas:

i) providing a medical laboratory that examines, organizes, represents and catalogue medical information and knowledge;

ii) producing technologically improved tools that provide support for medical decisions, training and research;

iii) integrating various activities in a medical/medical laboratory, computer science and other sciences that are necessary for the optimum function;

iv) offering a wider scope of learning in medical, MLS trainings and specializations.

SN	Equipment	Sample in use	Parameters
1	Glucometer	Blood/sensors	Glucose
2	Lipids/cholesterol meter	Blood	Cholesterol Triglycerides High-density lipoprotein
3	Automated hematology analyser	Whole blood	RBC, WBC, Hb, platelets, Blood differentials
4	Automated chemistry analyzers	Plasma/serum	All clinical chemistry parameters of interest
5	Blood culture machine	Blood	Microorganism growth Sensitivity of drugs
6	Semen analyzers	Semen	Sperm counts Motility Progression Other semen parameters

Table 2.1. *Some AI equipment and parameters of interest in medical laboratories*

2.4. Medical Laboratory Information Management System, centralized data and WWW

Data is very important for AI systems. The systems should be able to understand the patterns or characteristics from data in order to generate accurate and precise results. Modern AI methods use a large amount of medical data to interpret the patterns in data, examine data used in the training of system algorithms, and then apply them in real medical laboratory practice if trained method performance is acceptable (Goyal et al. 2021).

Medical data are grouped into unstructured and structured data. Data is said to be structured if it is well organized and can be analyzed by conventional computational methods, such as data mining and databases, or manually. They exist as databases with defined relationships specified by human experts. Unstructured data are neither directly analyzable nor standardized due to defects such as imprecision, noise, inconsistency and incompleteness (Goyal et al. 2021).

Computer vision and NLP often use different preprocessing methods to convert data into forms that are uniform and can be processed before applying AI methods (Goyal et al. 2021).

Today, digitalization, automation and laboratory information software are commonplace in clinical laboratories (Sisman and Basok 2020). A proposed model for web-based medical diagnosis and prediction has four components, which include diagnosis module, databases, prediction module and user interface. Prediction module uses neural network (NN) techniques to guess a patient's health conditions, based on past closely related cases (Shortliffe et al. 2000).

NN is a network of many simple processors or units. It has the capability to read a set of data and then construct weight matrices to symbolize the learning patterns (Sarle 1999). It simulates the activity of a human brain to execute tasks as a human does.

The databases include patient–disease and patients' databases. Patients' databases contain a patient's bio-data (like name and addresses), while patient–disease database stores all the patients' details, including their health problems (disease types and therapy). The user interface in the proposed model is the WWW for the users to interact with the systems. Data from the patients and patient–disease databases are used for training and testing (Shortliffe et al. 2000).

Centralized databases over the WWW make it possible for medical professionals from all over the world to collaborate, share information, knowledge and expertise, conduct online diagnosis and treatment of diseases, and have discussion online (Shortliffe et al. 1996). Another interactive medical diagnostic system that can be accessed online is the "Experienced Based Medical Diagnostics System" (Manickam and Abidi 1999). Fuzzy logic is applied in fuzzy relational reasoning for medical diagnosis. It deals with uncertainty in knowledge that assumes human reasoning in sketchy data (Shortliffe et al. 2000).

AI systems in medical applications are broadly grouped into two main types: machine learning (ML) and natural language processing (NLP). ML systems try to understand the potential disease effects or to get personal information or attributes of the patients, such as genetic information, imagery data and electric physiological (EP) data microscopic films, under the microscope and connected to computers. The NLP systems simplify structured health data by analyzing unstructured data (Health First Europe 2020), and generate organized records that are accessible to the system and can be analyzed by ML techniques (Gadde et al. 2020). This is applied in MLS, where improved and automated machines such as microscopes, sperm analyzers, hematology and chemical pathology analyzers that are linked to computers generate abundant data for analysis/processing and interpretation, and finally give a result that leads to improvement in patients' health.

2.5. Artificial intelligence methodologies and their application in medical laboratory science

Computer-aided diagnosis (CAD) involves the use of different AI technologies to detect and/or classify diseases with better accuracy, in the form of computer output (Goyal et al. 2021). According to the World Health Organization (WHO), about 1/6 deaths globally are due to cancer, and makes cancer the second leading cause of death. A lot of AI-based systems have been designed to automate prognosis of different classes of cancer. Computer-aided ML- or DL-based systems could assist in precise early-stage diagnosis and staging of cancer.

Swapna et al. (2018) proposed a hybrid DL-based model for diagnosis of diabetes mellitus (DM) that entails examination of the heart rate variability (HRV) signal obtained from the ECG signal dataset. Different machine learning (ML) statistical attributes were proposed by Santhanam and Padmavathi (2015) to automate the diagnosis of DM and was shown to be very successful in that regard (above 98% accuracy). These involved the use of the K-means clustering algorithm to remove noise (outliers), followed by the application of a genetic algorithm to extract the best set of features, which are then fed to SVM for classification. Other such ML statistical attributes proposed for the same purpose include KNN, random forest and J48 (Goyal et al. 2021).

Many studies and research have been published, which propose automated diagnosis of infectious diseases. Shen et al. (2016) proposed using blood cells image data for the diagnosis of malaria parasitic infection. Pasa et al. (2019) proposed computerized diagnosis of tuberculosis by the use of memory-prompt 25-layered deep CNN. Feller et al. (2018) proposed processing medical and clinical notes through NLP to assess the risk of HIV/AIDS. Examination of stained microscopic sputum images was proposed by Mithra and Emmanuel (2019) as an automated approach to detect and count bacilli. Using electronic health records (EHR) is proposed by Lauritsen et al. (2020) for the diagnosis of sepsis infection. Abdullah et al. (2018) evaluated and proposed MLP, SVM and KNN as proficient statistical ML classifiers for the automated diagnosis of hepatitis using hepatitis risk factor data repository. EHR is also proposed by Goyal et al. (2021) to classify skin infections and other diseases in healthcare.

In the presence of varicocele and male infertility, along with about one aberrant semen parameter, varicocele remediation is usually advisable. However, approximately 1:2 of men who meet these criteria for repair do not show productive results, despite successful treatment. Hence, an AI model was developed that can use R to predict the men with varicocele who could benefit from treatment and more likely upgrade after surgery (Jesse et al. 2022).

An AI-based image processing program is formulated to non-invasively measure the glucose concentration in a patient's urine sample and is used to deduce the equivalent concentration of glucose in blood. The technique is based on the principle of photometric analysis and gives the most precise glucose value in blood. Using conventional methods, diabetic patients usually monitor their glucose levels regularly, in which case, they prick the fingers at least four times a day to take blood samples for the test (Geetha and Lakshminarayanan 2013).

Elman recurrent artificial neural networks (ANNs) have been reported to be effective in predicting blood glucose levels (BGLs), which is based on a history of meal intake, BGLs and insulin shot. Devices such as continuous blood glucose meters (CGMs) and insulin pumps (IPs) are proposed to salvage the burden of BGL control on the patient (Robertson et al. 2011). Table 2.2 presents some research views (Aframian et al. 2020; Bharath 2021), based on AI applications in medical laboratories.

SN	Name	Full meaning	Section where in use
1	AI	Artificial Intelligence	All aspect of medical laboratories using digital machines and automations
2	ANN	Artificial Neural Network	Diagnosis of diabetes (sugar) and fats/oils (cholesterol) Liver and cardiac complications Brain and neuronal issues Cell population data
3	CASNET	Casual Association Networks	Diagnosis and treatment of diseases
4	CBR	Case-Based Reasoning	Automated diagnosis
5	CIG	Computer Interpretable Guidelines	Automated diagnosis Gestational diagnosis
6	DM	Data Mining	All sections of medical laboratory science and healthcare

7	DT	Decision Tress	Explanation of diagnosis, revealing the risk of cardiac- or cancer-related issues
8	ES	Expert Systems	Automated diagnosis
9	FL	Fuzzy Logic	Automated diagnosis Glucose and protein assays
10	GA	Genetic Algorithms	Diagnosis of diabetes (sugar) and fats/oils (cholesterol)
11	HERMES	Hepatology Rule-Based Medical Expert Systems	Prognosis of chronic liver diseases
12	ICTH	Intelligent Child Healthcare Treatment	Children diagnosis and mortality
13	ISS	Interactive STD Station	Diagnosis and data of STDs
14	ML	Machine Learning	Automated diagnosis
15	MLML	Medical Laboratory Machine Learning	Medical laboratory diagnosis, data and analytics
16	MLP	Multi-Layer Perception	Automated diagnosis
17	MSE	Mean Square Error	Automated diagnosis
18	MYCIN		Diagnosis of antimicrobials and sensitivity testing
19	PIP	Present Illness Program	Nephrological history and data/records
20	RBR	Rule-Based Reasoning	Diagnosis of diabetes (sugar) and fats/oils (cholesterol) Automated diagnosis
21	SVM	Support Vector Machine	Diagnosis of diabetes (sugar) and fats/oils (cholesterol)

Table 2.2. *Some AI applications of interest in medical laboratory diagnosis*

AI in MLS is well appreciated in automated systems. Automation in medical laboratory is a fast growing and innovative area, which involves the use of machines that will independently perform laboratory duties. This includes specimen collection, sample analysis and generation of results that are clinically valuable. They operate based on the basic principles of some traditional laboratory processes. They are important in economizing sample and reagent volumes to accommodate patients that are not able to provide high sample volumes for multiple tests. The majority of the automated medical laboratory machines have AI-based systems and programs that allow for easy, fast, efficient and independent processes, and generate accurate and precise results. Invariably, AI would not be fully implemented without adopting automation systems in various medical laboratories (Aframian et al. 2020).

2.6. Nigerian medical laboratory intelligence before, now and future

Although already at advanced levels and wider applications in medical laboratories in the developed countries (albeit, there is still room for much improvement), the application of AI is required in medical and diagnostic laboratories in Nigeria. At present, it is akin to virgin land; there is a moderate new approach to laboratory practice, with very few adopting one or two. Many laboratory physicians and medical laboratory personnel are yet to come to terms with the resolute quality, acceptability, application and how to coordinate the AI technologies into medical laboratory practice so that it would not undermine medical expertise (Gayathri et al. 2018).

Presently in Nigeria, computer technology is being applied to reduce time and cost during patient registration in the hospital/laboratory. A patient's record could be updated by simply entering the patient's ID by the front desk officers during patient visit to the hospital/laboratory. Signals are automatically sent to notify the physician and/or medical laboratory specialists who can refer to the patient's history record during sampling, diagnosis and a treatment history. Medical laboratory test results, once generated, could equally be sent automatically to the consulting physician and the patient. Drug prescription can also be sent automatically to the dispensary (Shortliffe et al. 2000) with a good medical laboratory information management system (MLIMS) (Obeta et al. 2022a).

AI is a high-tech creation and adapts to the change of the modern era. It therefore follows the trend of time as the fateful outcome of the progress in science and technology. AI technology is playing a critical role in medical education, medical patient management and drug production, and has taken them into a new direction (Liu et al. 2021).

The future of the medical laboratory is that the laboratory professionals will be supported with AI. This will assist in supplementing human experience, wisdom and knowledge. AI and ML software are already integrating themselves as tools to enhance accuracy and efficiency in a medical laboratory. Prominent educational organizations or hospital/research laboratories and start-up companies are working seriously in collaboration to develop software that will address different disease conditions, especially cancer (Menon 2020).

However, the future of AI in medical laboratory diagnosis in Nigeria seems scary. There is growing evidence that the traditional method of medical care by some medical professionals is being diverted to the use of AI chatbots. This is the AI version of some healthcare providers. The application of AI in medical laboratory diagnosis is evolving and growing fast through the field of ML and Big Data analytics (Gayathri et al. 2018). The future of AI is already here, and the revolution is expected to be fast and could take Nigerian medical laboratories into an unprecedented era (Liu et al. 2021).

2.7. Medical laboratory services where AI is used in Nigeria

MLS, although with numerous nomenclatures across the globe (Obeta et al. 2020), is the profession that deals with the analysis of human specimens for accurate diagnosis of ailments and possible drugs of choice, especially in susceptibility testing (Obeta et al. 2019a, 2019b). Successfully, Covid-19 has brought an advancement in medical laboratory practice in Nigeria, leading to various upgrading of facilities, equipment and services (Obeta et al. 2021). This digital era commenced in medical laboratories that encourage MLAI.

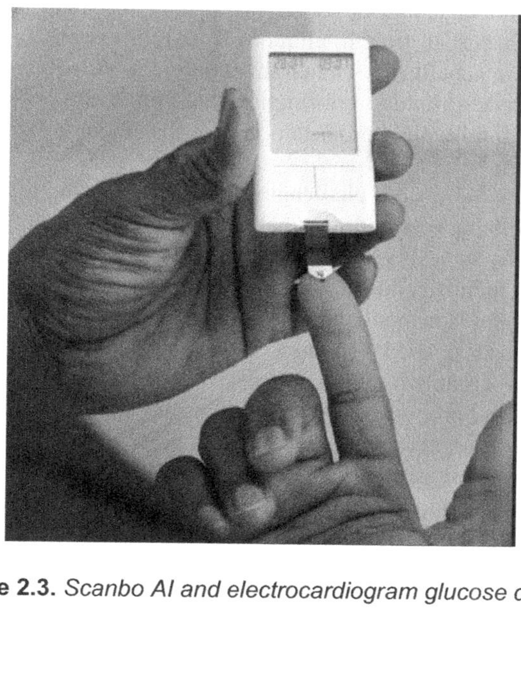

Figure 2.3. *Scanbo AI and electrocardiogram glucose device*

Urinalysis is a basic diagnostic test performed to ascertain pathological changes in the analytes found in urine. The conventional urine dipstick test is to immerse the test strip briefly in a well-mixed urine sample and observe the strip visually for any color change. The results analyzed in such a way were prone to bias or human errors due to visual problems (Huchegowda et al. 2021; Tan et al. 2021). With the advent of AI, there have been improvements in the way urinalysis is performed, following the development of AI-based POCT urine analyzers, which read the strips and give approximate values of the analytes in the urine being analyzed. This solves the problem and helps both the laboratory professional and the patient to get more accurate, reliable and faster results. Many Nigerian medical laboratories are adopting this new technology in their operations, especially POCT glucose meter using AI and electrocardiogram, as shown in Figure 2.3, which uses photoplethysmogram.

Blood culture is used to detect sepsis (bloodstream infections (BSIs)) and identify the causative organisms. Sepsis is one of the leading causes of death globally (Pai et al. 2021). Early detection and commencement of effective treatment is very important to ensure successful treatment of the infection. The traditional blood culture method is time-consuming because of the many steps needed to identify the pathogens (Wisplinghoff et al. 2004). In addition, there are usually delays in antibiotic testing and the administration of effective drugs. This could increase the patient's risk of death (Schwaber and Carmeli 2007). A patient's blood sample is usually inoculated in broth for pre-culture to detect bacterial growth, if present. If there is bacterial growth, aliquot of the broth is obtained to make smear for Gram stain and to subculture. The Gram stain gives a clue about the implicating organism and the first evaluative information that guides the physician on the most appropriate therapy to initiate in order to optimize the outcome (Smith et al. 2018).

To address the associated challenges with the conventional blood culture method, effective biomarkers and automated AI-based blood culture systems have been developed to detect BSIs early (Pai et al. 2021). These are ML models powered by AI for the early identification of patients with a high risk of BSIs, especially in the ICU. Automated image acquisition and convolutional neural network (CNN)-based approach is used for automated Gram stain image interpretation and classification of the organism. There are also two models, logistic regression and gradient boosted trees, proposed to promptly predict bacteremia in patients. Using the NN model, an ML approach has the ability to predict positive blood culture with high specificity but low sensitivity (Mahmoud et al. 2021). This may be beneficial in reducing unnecessary blood cultures and the associated additional costs (Boerman et al. 2022). Although some hospitals and laboratories in Nigeria have adopted this automated blood culture system, the majority of the Nigerian laboratories still depend on the conventional methods.

Complete blood count (CBC), also known as full blood count (FBC), is one of the fundamental tests performed to assess overall health and various disease conditions of a patient, including hematological abnormalities. It gives approximate values (cell population data (CPD)) of the different blood cell types and red cell indices of a given patient blood sample. This produces varied blood cell parameters used to diagnose different types of diseases (Alam and Islam 2019; Shabbir et al. 2020). Conventionally, manual counting of blood cells is done using a hemocytometer (counting chamber) and microscope after staining with appropriate stains. This is time-consuming and stressful. Data analytics using ML algorithms, such as ANN models, is used to screen hematological malignancies using CPD. This appears to be an efficient tool for medical laboratory testing of hematological malignancies. This plays a crucial role in revolutionizing medical laboratory diagnostics. Another ML approach to automatically identify and count RBCs, WBCs and platelets is the "you only look once" (YOLO) object detection and classification algorithm. This uses a method-based IOU and KNN to avoid counting of the same object more than once with high accuracy (Alam and Islam 2019). Many big Nigerian medical laboratories are already using fully automated hematology analyzers for FBC.

Conventionally, semen analysis in the medical laboratories depends mainly on a manual microscopy technique. The technique is tedious, time-consuming, laboratory-based and prejudiced. This led to the development of the "computer-assisted semen analyzers (CASAs)" for semi-automated routine analysis of semen, which also had the problem of complicated operation and not being widely accepted; this has been in use in Nigerian medical laboratories like Abims Fertility and Garmete Banking Services Lagos, Nigeria (Figure 2.4).

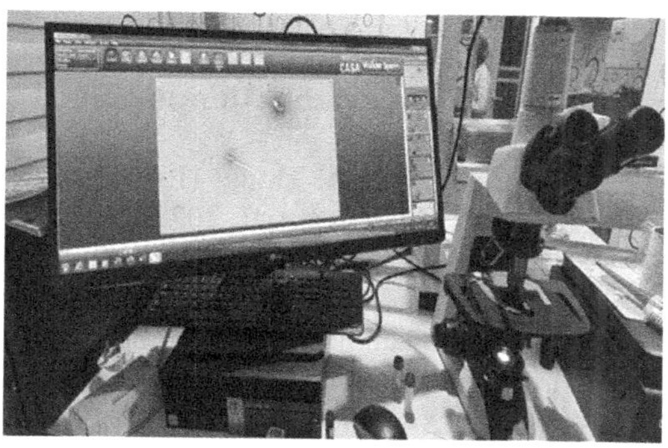

Figure 2.4. *Computer-assisted semen analyzers (CASAs) in use in Nigeria*

A novel, automated, artificial intelligence optical microscopic (AIOM)-based technology, LensHooke™ X1 PRO (X1 PRO) (Figure 2.5), has been designed and developed for sperm quality analysis. It is an accessible, rapid and standardized method for quantitative measurement of sperm concentration, motility and seminal pH. It is based on an in-built high-resolution and autofocus optical lens in combination with an AI auto-calculation system (Agarwal et al. 2019).

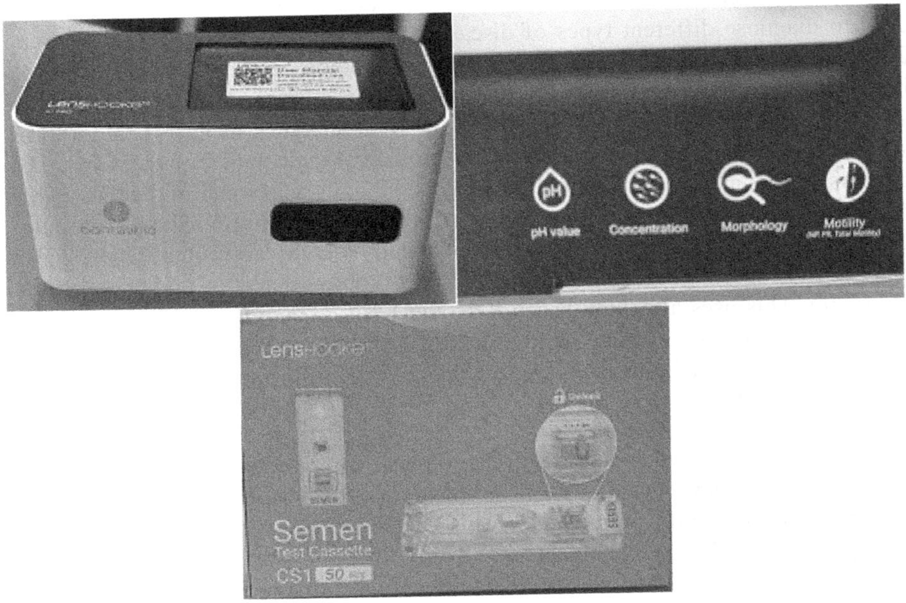

Figure 2.5. *AI semen analysis machine, parts and accessories (LensHooke™) in use in Lagos, Nigeria*

2.8. AI and Internet of medical laboratory things

The integration of AI and the Internet of Things (IoT), also called the Internet of medical laboratory things (IoMLTs) (Obeta et al. 2022b), is one of the three major modes or means by which medical laboratories and hospitals can apply the AI technologies to monitor patients' compliance to instructions about adequate preparation and fasting prior to sampling, and compliance to the prescribed treatment regimen and improved clinical outcomes (Gadde et al. 2020).

The integration of AI and IoMLTs gives an opportunity for online assessment, diagnosis and transmission of results to patients and other medical laboratory clients within and outside of the medical laboratory facility. AI and IoMLTs are a trending development in Medical Laboratory Services that should be encouraged in developing nations such as Nigeria.

Greaves et al. (2019) analyzed AI techniques for web-based medical applications and proposed a model for web-based medical diagnosis and predictions (Shortliffe et al. 2000). Nigeria remains a virgin land where such gadgets and equipment could be well accommodated and used as the majority of laboratory facilities are yet to acquire them.

2.9. Opportunities and challenges of AI for Nigerian medical laboratories

AI-based systems have revolutionized medical laboratory practice in modern days globally and the Nigerian medical laboratories are not left out. The advantages and opportunities that come with it cannot be overemphasized. They assist and guide the human professionals in their practice in many ways. The ease with which laboratory personnel can access real-time data today offers great opportunities for disease prevention, early diagnosis and treatment (Sisman and Basok 2020). However, while AI is being accepted positively, the applications in medical laboratories come with both the "utopian perspective" (new opportunities) and the "dystopian view" (challenges to overcome) (Lee and Yoon 2021). The Nigerian medical laboratories have become endangered species laboratories due to lack of political will to support them, inter-professional rivalries, quackery, poor implementation of medical laboratory policies, demotivated professionals and little interest from the management for further training and specializations of skills among medical laboratory professionals.

The advantages and opportunities of AI that could help Nigerian laboratories include the following:

– **Automation**: by using AI-based systems, it is possible to streamline diagnostic processes by obtaining reasonable data from a large number of patients, which give more insight to accurately predict the disease condition and enhance early detection of diseases (Mittal et al. 2020). Automation and AI systems have made it possible for hospital and stand-alone medical laboratories in Nigeria to expand their capacity to handle large patient inflow. AI in medical laboratory saves a lot of time and effort for the laboratory personnel that they spend on manual processes and test reports. The Nigerian laboratories should move further from manual and semi-automated practice to AI-based automations. This would expand the scope and improve the quality of services provided.

– **Efficiency**: AI-based systems can understand, diagnose and efficiently predict disease faster; it is also cost-effective (Ejaz et al. 2018). The application of computational approach enhances (improves) interpretation of medical laboratory reports and further increases the potency of laboratory diagnostics in the process of patient management and clinical judgment (Sisman and Basok 2020). This efficiency, when AI systems are fully in use in Nigeria, would encourage an increase in accredited facilities and equally improve medical laboratory services.

– **Accuracy**: with the AI systems, laboratory results generated are more accurate and precise, since they are devoid of errors and bias associated with humans. This provides opportunity for effective laboratory quality and management systems (Javed et al. 2019). AI uses step-wise algorithms to analyze large datasets in medical care, and the results are used to make a decision to assist in medical diagnosis of diseases. The AI systems have the ability to learn and correct themselves to improve their accuracy (Goyal et al. 2021). AI-based systems also have the ability to give out results quickly and can change the unproductive conventional medical laboratory model that cannot give timely and accurate resolutions in the cases of complicated diagnoses (Liu et al. 2021). The accuracy provided by AI systems could reduce the mortality rate in Nigeria and encourage adequate diagnosis and clinical management.

– **Handling large and difficult data**: AI-based algorithms can handle, process and analyze large complex data that are difficult for human experts to perform. The systems can use results from the analysis to recommend the right treatment (Shortliffe et al. 2000; Goyal et al. 2021). Given Nigeria's large population, there is no doubt that AI-based systems serve the best for Nigerian medical laboratories.

– **Decision support system**: AI-based systems make processes such as managing resource allocation and patient inflow seamless and timely, coupled with proper disease diagnosis and analysis (Goyal et al. 2021).

– **AI for research and specialization**: with the advent of AI-based systems in medical laboratory practice, doors have opened to new research areas and specialization for scientists interested in developing new skills and expertise in innovative algorithms to increase the efficiency of different medical laboratory processes being solved via AI (Rehman 2020). AI-based technologies have provided many possibilities for innovation in the knowledge-intensive medical and research laboratories (Shortliffe et al. 2000; Lee and Yoon 2021). Such research and specializations are much needed in Nigerian medical laboratories as AI could be the needed systems.

The speedy improvement of information technologies (ITs) will increase the consultancy function of medical laboratories by facilitating the control of POCT analyzers and direct contact with patients (Sisman and Basok 2020).

2.10. Risks/limitations and challenges associated with AI in Nigerian medical laboratories

Despite the numerous benefits and opportunities associated with the AI technology, the application of AI in medical laboratory practice is faced with limitations and challenges (Goyal et al. 2021), some of which are discussed below:

– **Error in medical diagnosis**: the development of AI in medical laboratory systems needs specialized programmers with knowledge of both areas of computer language programming and medical laboratory, which at present are not readily available. This makes it difficult to adequately design specialized AI-based medical laboratory systems. In Nigeria, overdependence on these systems can lead to diagnostic errors (Goyal et al. 2021; Lee and Yoon 2021). However, the errors seen in manual practice are worse than anticipated errors from AI systems.

– **Need for expertise training and slow adaptation**: to fully apply AI in the different medical laboratory processes, training and retraining of medical laboratory personnel and professional realignment is required. This is usually faced with low enthusiasm and slow adaptation to the new systems among the medical laboratory practitioners in Nigeria, who are already used to the manual and analogue systems, limited knowledge and poor confidence about the abilities of the AI systems (Goyal et al. 2021). The need for expertise training fully supported by management and enthusiasm for change is key to better medical laboratory practice in Nigeria.

– **High cost**: one of the major challenges facing the application of AI in Nigerian medical laboratories is the high cost to purchase, install and maintain the systems. The majority of the AI-based systems require steady power and Internet access to function optimally and update the software automatically, the absence of which may lead to system failure. The high cost makes it difficult (or impossible) for most Nigerian medical laboratories to adopt the AI-based processes (Goyal et al. 2021). In particular, the advantages of AI systems outweigh the cost implications that militate against the order of the machines. The AI systems should be procured by various authorities in Nigerian medical laboratories, not minding the high cost for the better laboratory service in Nigeria.

– **Ethical standards and data privacy**: the use of AI systems can allow unauthorized persons to access confidential, private patient data. People may feel reluctant to give their data and tests using AI methods because there are no privacy standards and data protection. Inappropriate access to patients' data may put them at risk (Goyal et al. 2021; Lee and Yoon 2021). Although this limits the attention to AI systems, policies and security software are necessary for better use in Nigeria.

– **Performance standards and rush in AI deployment**: the medical laboratories in Nigeria have observed a speedy attitude in deploying AI-based automated systems in laboratories in order to make more money without relevant gradual testing, training and validation. This rush has led to system failure (Goyal et al. 2021). There is a need to formulate standards for measuring the performance of AI systems quantitatively (Majid et al. 2020), and such advancement should be encouraged in Nigerian medical laboratories.

2.11. AI and digitalization of Nigerian medical laboratories

In digitized organizations, information and communication technology (ICT) is an integral component needed to enhance competitive advantage and facilitate operational potency (Lee and Yoon 2021). In developed economies, hospitals and clinical laboratories are rapidly deploying digital technologies (Big Data analytics, AI, ML, Internet of Medical Laboratory Things (IoMLTs), and smart sensors and robots) in their services to ensure operational efficiency and better quality (Lee 2019; Obeta et al. 2022b). ML algorithms can be learned over a period of time without being specifically programmed (Rigla et al. 2018) and cannot be ignored in Nigerian medical laboratory as well.

The application of AI, Big Data and data science in the various laboratory processes can genuinely improve patients' experience throughout the whole healthcare system, ranging from disease prevention, screening, early diagnosis, treatment and management (Gruson 2021; Obeta et al. 2022a). The Covid-19 experience in Nigeria has explained it all; there is no doubt that AI systems and diagnostics of Nigerian medical laboratories are the way to go.

Effective applications of AI in Nigerian medical laboratories require proper planning and strategies to modify the entire laboratory services and operations in order to benefit from what the technologies can offer (Lee and Yoon 2021).

It is expected that Nigerian medical laboratories in this digital era, according to (Sisman and Basok 2020), should work towards focusing on the following: implementation of a total quality management system (TQMS), the test value and not the test volume, effective diagnostic management, medical laboratory equipment operational efficiency, medical laboratory staff and patient safety, risk management, consolidation of conventional tests, quality assurance and quality control, reduction in medical laboratory errors, reduction in number of inappropriate test requests, following the global standardization of tests, consolidation on the routine tests, development of new tests, adequate management of POCT and the instruments, new technology acceptance, more staff training, verification of test interpretation algorithms, and adequate storage of medical laboratory information in one place.

2.12. Conclusion

The progress in computer technology has boosted the development of software to assist clinicians in clinical judgment without direct interactions with the medical laboratory specialists. The software development uses the latent feature of human intelligence (making decisions, reasoning and learning by experience). The software was developed to assist medical professionals in diagnosis and predict patient's condition based on certain rules or "experience", not meant to replace the specialist. Computer technology could be applied for better patient management and to reduce the patient's waiting time to see the medical laboratory specialist, and to reduce mortality rate (Shortliffe et al. 2000). The current copiousness of health data is leading the way to a transformation from the analytical ability in diagnostic tests to the cognition to integrate data; and at the same time, interpret them within the clinical context (Sisman and Basok 2020).

Although many medical laboratory processes are still being done manually or partly automated in Nigeria, there are concerted efforts and research ongoing to improve the pre-analytic, analytic and post-analytic medical laboratory processes with AI-support. These AI-supported systems are intended to predict a patient's wait time in the phlebotomy unit, organize the process of blood collection or the auto-verification of test results with the ML approach (Orbatu et al. 2020); this is so the challenges of the past and present (Badnjević et al. 2021; Paranjape et al. 2021), especially in Nigeria, can be better placed for the future.

The ML approach can also be programmed to ascertain similarities between analyzers in key laboratories where various instruments that run the same analytes are tested and/or monitored to predict and detect equipment failures before they occur (Sisman and Basok 2020). AI can also assist medical laboratory professionals on how to correct a problem or to improve a medical and diagnostic process.

Medical laboratories could play an active role in the future as a "nerve center of diagnostics" and joining the patient and physician in forming a "Diagnostics 4.0" triangle. The AI, MLIMS, IoMLTs, MLIMS and other technological-driven packages should be incorporated into various medical laboratories, including Nigerian medical laboratories, for better quality services for the patients and entire healthcare facilities, just as it experienced during Covid-19 (Akbar 2022).

Medical laboratory specialists in Nigeria could become cardinal actors in the process of expeditious and risk-free integration of Big Data and AI technologies to healthcare, and in the grooming of manpower and counselling of patients; this, in the long run, could have a remarkable socio-economic advantage on the healthcare systems in Nigeria (Gruson 2021).

Despite the numerous advantages and opportunities associated with the application of AI in medical laboratories, it is also faced with lots of challenges. The software components with the ability to learn without human management can act in unexpected ways. They may deviate from social norms due to the use of inadequate parameters in their design. Such deviation may lead to irretrievable failure. There is therefore the need for constant monitoring by humans (Goyal et al. 2021), must be used with care and attention.

There is a fear among medical laboratory professionals that they will be replaced by AI systems. Reassurance is required that AI systems are there to help, not to replace them (Majid et al. 2020).

To encourage the digitization and maximum application of AI in Nigerian medical laboratories, it is recommended that "computational medical laboratory" units be constituted and integrated into postgraduate and undergraduate education curricula. There is a great need to keep the systems and laboratories where AI is applied updated with recent developments (Goyal et al. 2021).

Medical laboratory management and/or instrumentation and fabrication department/faculty of the Federal School of Medical Laboratory Science Jos/West Africa Postgraduate College of Medical Laboratory Science is the right place to domicile the prospective trainees of AI, Automation, MLAI, IoMLTs, MLIMS and the technological improvement of medical laboratory perspectives in Nigeria, and the world at large.

2.13. References

Abdullah, H.N., Abd, B.H., Muhi, S.H. (2018). High-resolution systems for automated diagnosis of hepatitis. *2018 Third Scientific Conference of Electrical Engineering (SCEE)*, 39–44. doi: 10.1109/SCEE.2018.8684154.

Aframian, A., Iranpour, F., Cobb, J. (2020). Medical devices and artificial intelligence. In *Artificial Intelligence in Healthcare*, Bohr, A. and Memarzadeh, K. (eds). Academic Press, 163–177. doi: 10.1016/B978-0-12-818438-7.00007-1.

Agarwal, A., Henkel, R., Huang, C.C., Lee, M.S. (2019). Automation of human semen analysis using a novel artificial intelligence optical microscopic technology. *Andrologia*, e13440. doi: 10.1111/and.13440.

Akbar, K. (2022). Artificial intelligence apps for COVID-19 virus. *Acad. Lett.*, Article 4845. doi: 10.20935/AL4845.

Alam, M.M. and Islam, M.T. (2019). Machine learning approach of automatic identification and counting of blood cells. *Healthcare Technol. Lett.*, 6(4), 103–108. doi: 10.1049/htl.2018.5098.

Badnjević, A., Halida Avdihodžić, H., Pokvić, L.G. (2021). Artificial intelligence in medical devices: Past, present and future. *Science, Art & Religion*, 1(1–2), 101–106.

Bharath, A.A. (2021). Recent advancements in AI – implications for medical device technology and certification. BSI [Online]. Available at: https://www.bsigroup.com/globalassets/meddev/localfiles/en-us/whitepapers/bsi-md-ai-whitepaper.pdf.

Boerman, A.W., Schinkel, M., Meijerink, L., van den Ende, E.S., Pladet, L.C.A., Scholtemeijer, M.G., Zeeuw, J., van der Zaag, A.Y., Minderhoud, T.C., Elbers, P.W.G. et al. (2022). Using machine learning to predict blood culture outcomes in the emergency department: A single-centre, retrospective, observational study. *BMJ Open*, 12, e053332. doi: 10.1136/bmjopen-2021-053332.

Ceriotti, F. (2019). Is there a classical role for the clinical laboratory in digital health? *Clin. Chem. Lab. Med.*, 57(3), 353–358.

Delipetrev, B., Tsinarakii, C., Kostić, U. (2020). Historical evolution of artificial intelligence. EUR 30221 EN. Publications Office of the European Union, Luxembourg. doi: 10.2760/801580JRC120469.

Ejaz, K., Rahim, M.S.M., Rehman, A., Chaudhry, H., Saba, T., Ejaz, A., Ej, C.F. (2018). Segmentation method for pathological brain tumor and accurate detection using MRI. *Int. J. Adv. Comput. Sci. Appl.*, 9(8), 394–401.

Etukudoh, N.S. and Obeta, M.U. (2021). Patients' (clients) satisfaction with medical laboratory services contributes to health and quality improvement. In *Healthcare Access*, Agrawal, A. and Kosgi, S. (eds). IntechOpen. doi: 10.5772/intechopen.99290.

Etukudoh, N.S., Nelson, A.B., Obeta, M.U., Ejinaka, O.R., Ibanga, I.E., Nwapi, L.L., Samuel, P. (2021). Health care delivery business and the role of Medical Laboratory Scientists. *IAR J. Med. Sci.*, 2(4), 76–80.

Feller, D.J., Zucker, J., Yin, M.T., Gordon, P., Elhadad, N. (2018). Using clinical notes and natural language processing for automated HIV risk assessment. *J. Acquir. Immune Defic. Syndr.*, 77(2), 160–166. doi: 10.1097/QAI.0000000000001580.

Gadde, S.S., Dinesh, V., Kalli, R. (2020). Applications of artificial intelligence in medical devices and healthcare. *Int. J. Comput. Sci. Trends Technol.*, 8(2), 182–188.

Gayathri, P., Gopichand, G., Amali, G.B., Santhi, H. (2018). A case study on artificial intelligence application in medical diagnostics. *World Wide J. Multidiscip. Res. Dev.*, 4(12), 100–103.

Geetha, S. and Lakshminarayanan, V. (2013). An artificial intelligence based glucometer for diabetic patients using urinal analysis. *Bonfring Int. J. Power Syst. Integr. Circuits*, 3(1), 1–6.

Goyal, L.M., Saba, T., Rehman, A., Larabi, S. (2021). *Artificial Intelligence and Internet of Things: Applications in Smart Healthcare*. CRC Press, Boca Raton.

Greaves, R.F., Bernardini, S., Ferrari, M., Fortina, P., Gouget, B., Gruson, D. (2019). Key questions about the future of laboratory medicine in the next decade of the 21st century: A report from the IFCC-Emerging Technologies Division. *Clin. Chim. Acta.*, 495, 570–589.

Gruson, D. (2021). Big data, artificial intelligence and laboratory medicine: Time for integration. *Adv. Lab. Med.*, 2(1), 1–3. doi: 10.1515/almed-2021-0003.

Health First Europe (2020). COMPENDIUM: Artificial intelligence in healthcare [Online]. Available at: https://healthfirsteurope.eu/publication/compendium-artificial-intelligence-in-healthcare/ [Accessed 30 March 2022].

Huchegowda, C., Huchegowda, R., Jain, J.B. (2021). Artificial intelligence based point-of-care test device for urinary dipstick analysis for urinary tract infection. *MJPS*, 7(1), 87–90.

Hussain, W., Ishak, W., Siraj, F. (2008). Artificial intelligence in medical application: An exploration. [Online]. Available at: https://www.academia.edu [Accessed 8 December 2023].

Hussein, B.R., Halimu C., Siddique, M.T (2020). The future of artificial intelligence and its social, economic and ethical consequences. *International Conference on Advances in Computing and Technology (ICACT–2020) Proceedings*.

Islam, M.M., Poly, T.N., Yang, H.C., Li, Y.C. (2021). Deep into laboratory: An artificial intelligence approach to recommend laboratory tests. *Diagnostics*, 11, 990. doi: 10.3390/diagnostics11060990.

Javed, R., Rahim, M.S.M., Saba, T. (2019). An improved framework by mapping salient features for skin lesion detection and classification using the optimized hybrid features. *Int. J. Adv. Trends Comput. Sci. Eng.*, 8(1), 95–101.

Jesse, O.M.B., Tradewell, U.B., Thiago, F.L., Sirpi, N., Daniel, C.G., Elie, N., Joseph, M., Vinayak, M., Lau, S., Jarvi, K. (2022). Artificial intelligence based machine learning models predict sperm parameter upgrading after varicocele repair: A multi-institutional analysis. *World J. Mens Health*, 40(4), 618–626. doi: 10.5534/wjmh.210159.

Lauritsen, S.M., Kalør, M.E., Kongsgaard, E.L., Lauritsen, K.M., Jørgensen, M.J., Lange, J., Thiesson, B. (2020). Early detection of sepsis utilizing deep learning on electronic health record event sequences. *Artificial Intelligence in Medicine*, 104, 101820.

LeCun, Y., Bengio, Y., Hinton, G. (2015). Deep learning. *Nature*, 521(7553), 436–444.

Lee, D.H. (2019). Effects of key value co-creation elements in the healthcare system: Focusing on technology applications. *Serv. Bus.*, 13, 389–417.

Lee, D.H. and Yoon, S.N. (2021). Application of artificial intelligence-based technologies in the healthcare industry: Opportunities and challenges. *Int. J. Environ. Res. Public Health*, 18, 271. doi: 10.3390/ijerph18010271.

Liu, P., Lu, L., Zhang, J., Huo, T., Liu, S., Ye, Z. (2021). Application of artificial intelligence in medicine: An overview. *Curr. Med. Sci.*, doi: 10.1007/s11596-021-2474-3.

Mahmoud, E., Dhoayan, M.A., Bosaeed, M., Johani, S.A., Yaseen, M., Arabi Y.M. (2021). Developing machine-learning prediction algorithm for bacteremia in admitted patients. *Infect. Drug Resistance*, 14, 757–765.

Majid, A., Khan, M.A., Yasmin, M., Rehman, A., Yousafzai, A., Tariq, U. (2020). Classification of stomach infections: A paradigm of convolutional neural network along with classical features fusion and selection. *Microsc. Res. Tech.*, 83(5), 562–576.

Manickam, S. and Abidi, S.S.R. (1999). Experienced based medical diagnostics system over the world wide web (WWW). *Proceedings of The First National Conference on Artificial Intelligence Application in Industry*, Kuala Lumpur, 47–56.

Menon, P.K. (2020). Effect of artificial intelligence in the clinical laboratory. *Medlab* [Online]. Available at: https://www.medlabme.com/magazine/en/Issue/2018-issue-21/effect-of-artificial-intelligence-in-clinical-laboratory.html.

Mithra, K.S. and Emmanuel, W.S. (2019). Automated identification of mycobacterium bacillus from sputum images for tuberculosis diagnosis. *Signal, Image and Video Processing*, 13(8), 1585–1592.

Mittal, A., Kumar, D., Mittal, M., Saba, T., Abunadi, I., Rehman, A., Roy, S. (2020). Detecting pneumonia using convolutions and dynamic capsule routing for chest X-ray images. *Sensors*, 20(4), 1068.

Obeta, M.U., Eze, E.M., Ofojekwu, M.N., Jwanse, R.I., Maduka, M.K. (2019a). Organogram for medical laboratory services in Nigerian Public Health Institutions. *North Am. Acad. Res.*, 2(6), 69–75. doi: 10.5281/zenodo.3246909.

Obeta, M.U., Maduka, K.M., Ofor, I.B., Ofojekwu, N.M. (2019b). Improving quality and cost diminution in modern healthcare delivery: The role of the medical laboratory scientists in Nigeria. *Int. J. Bus. Manage. Invention (IJBMI)*, 8(3), 8–19.

Obeta, M.U., Maduka, M.K., Ejinaka, O.R. (2020). Medical laboratory science; the distortion of nomenclature across the globe. *NZ J. Med. Lab. Sci.*, 74(1), 52.

Obeta, M.U, Nkereuwem, S,E., Okoli, C.C. (2021). Nigerian medical laboratory diagnosis of COVID-19; from grass to grace. In *Intelligent Computing Applications for COVID-19: Predictions, Diagnosis, and Prevention*, Saba, T. and Khan, A.R. (eds). CRC Press Taylor and Francis Group. 84–93. doi: 10.1201/9781003141105-5.

Obeta, U.M., Ejinaka, O.R., Etukudoh, N.S. (2022a). Data mining in medical laboratory service improves disease surveillance and quality healthcare. In *Prognostic Models in Healthcare: AI and Statistical Approaches, Studies in Big Data 109*, Saba, T., Rehman, A., Roy, S. (eds). doi: 10.1007/978-981-19-2057-8_17.

Obeta, M.U., Ibrahim, A.U., Ibanga, I.E., Okey-Orji, V.N., Ezeama, C.J., Ejinaka, O.R. (2022b). Acceptability of internet of medical laboratory things among female medical laboratory professionals in Jos-Nigeria. *Fifth International Conference of Women in Data Science (WiDS) at Prince Sultan University*, Riyadh, 28–29. doi: 10.1109/WiDS-PSU54548.2022.00026.

Orbatu, D., Yıldırım, O., Yaşar, E., Şişman, A.R., Sevinç, S. (2020). Patient wait times in the phlebotomy unit. *Glob. J. Med. Res.*, 1.

Pai, K.C., Wang, M.S., Chen, Y.F., Tseng, C.H., Liu, P.Y., Chen, L.C., Sheu, R.K., Wu, C.L. (2021). An artificial intelligence approach to bloodstream infections prediction. *J. Clin. Med.*, 10, 2901. doi: 10.3390/jcm10132901.

Paranjape, K., Schinkel, M., Hammer, R.D., Schouten, B.O., Panday, R.S.N., Elbers, P.W.G., Kramer, M.H.H., Prabath Nanayakkara, P. (2021). The value of artificial intelligence in laboratory medicine current opinions and barriers to implementation. *Am. J. Clin. Pathol.*, 155, 823–831. doi: 10.1093/AJCP/AQAA170.

Pasa, F., Golkov, V., Pfeiffer, F., Cremers, D., Pfeiffer, D. (2019). Efficient deep network architectures for fast chest X-ray tuberculosis screening & visualization. *Sci. Rep.*, 9(1), 1–9.

Rehman, A. (2020). An ensemble of neural networks for nonlinear segmentation of over-lapped cursive script. *Int. J. Comput. Vis. Robot.*, 10(4), 275–288.

Rigla, M., García-Sáez, G., Pons, B., Hernando, M.E. (2018). Artificial intelligence methodologies and their application to diabetes. *Journal of Diabetes Science and Technology*, 12(2) 303–310. doi: 10.1177/1932296817710475.

Robertson, G., Lehmann, E.D., Sandham, W., Hamilton, D. (2011). Blood glucose prediction using artificial neural networks trained with the AIDA diabetes simulator: A proof-of-concept pilot study. *J. Electr. Comput. Eng.*, Article ID 681786. doi: 10.1155/2011/681786.

Safavi, K. and Kalis, B. (2019). How AI can change the future of health care. *Harv. Bus. Rev.*, [Online]. Available at: https://hbr.org/webinar/2019/02/how-ai-can-change-the-future-of-health-care [Accessed 30 August 22].

Santhanam, T. and Padmavathi, M.S. (2015). Application of K-means and genetic algorithms for dimension reduction by integrating SVM for diabetes diagnosis. *Procedia Comput. Sci.*, 47, 76–83.

Sarle, W.S. (1999). Neural Network FAQ, part 1 of 7: Introduction. Periodic posting to the Usenet Newsgroup comp.ai.neural-nets [Online]. Available at: ftp://ftp.sas.com/pub/neurl/FAQ.html.

Schwaber, M.J. and Carmeli, Y. (2007). Mortality and delay in effective therapy associated with extended-spectrum beta-lactamase production in *Enterobacteriaceae bacteraemia*: A systematic review and meta-analysis. *J. Antimicrob. Chemother.*, 60, 913–920. doi: 10.1093/jac/dkm318.

Shabbir, S.A., Firdani, R.P., Chung, H.J., Uddin, M., Hur, M., Park, J.H., Kim, H.W., Gradišek, A., Dovgan, E. (2020). Artificial intelligence based models for screening of hematologic malignancies using cell population data. *Sci. Rep.*, 10, 4583. doi: 10.1038/s41598-020-61247-0.

Shen, H., Pan, W.D., Dong, Y., Alim, M. (2016). Lossless compression of curated erythrocyte images using deep autoencoders for malaria infection diagnosis. *Picture Coding Symposium (PCS)*, 1–5. doi: 10.1109/PCS.2016.7906393.

Shortliffe, E.H., Barnet, G.O., Cimino, J.J., Greenes, R.A, Huff, S.M. Patel, V.L. (1996). Collaborative medical informatics research using the internet and the world wide web. *Proceedings of the AMIA Annual Fall Symposium*, Washington, DC, 125–129.

Shortliffe, E.H., Fagan, L.M., Yu, V.L. (2000). The infectious diseases physician and the Internet. In *Mandell, Douglas, and Bennett's Principles and Practice of Infectious Diseases*, Mandell, G.L., Bennett, J.E., Dolin, R. (eds). Churchill Livingstone, Inc., Pennsylvania, 3258–3263.

Sisman, A.R. and Basok, B.I. (2020). Digitalization and artificial intelligence in laboratory medicine. *Int. J. Med. Biochem.*, 3(2), 106–110. doi: 10.14744/ijmb.2020.81994.

Smith, K.P., Kang, A.D., Kirby, J.E. (2018). Automated interpretation of blood culture Gram stains by use of a deep convolutional neural network. *J. Clin. Microbiol.*, 56, e01521-17. doi: 10.1128/JCM.01521-17.

Swapna, G., Vinayakumar, R., Soman, K.P. (2018). Diabetes detection using deep learning algorithms. *ICT Express*, 4(4), 243–246.

Tan, J., Qin, F., Yuan, J. (2021). Current applications of artificial intelligence combined with urine detection in disease diagnosis and treatment. *Transl. Androl. Urol.*, 10(4), 1769–1779. doi: 10.21037/tau-20-1405.

Wisplinghoff, H., Bischoff, T., Tallent, S.M., Seifert, H., Wenzel, R.P., Edmond, M.B. (2004). Nosocomial bloodstream infections in US hospitals: Analysis of 24,179 cases from a prospective nationwide surveillance study. *Clin. Infect. Dis.*, 39, 309–317. doi: 10.1086/421946.

3

Machine Learning and Deep Learning for Smart City Services

Significant problems have emerged in metropolitan settings, such as traffic congestion, air pollution, energy use and public safety concerns. Many of these issues have been addressed intelligently and integrated by the Internet of Things (IoT) solutions. Due to the rapid advancement of IoT technology, researchers are driven to develop complex applications that take advantage of massive amounts of data provided by IoT-based devices/sensors. The use of in-depth learning (DL) and machine learning (ML) methodologies and urban development produced models such as climate, preparation, monitoring and investigation of the intelligence of intelligent cities. The application of ML and deep learning in the construction of smart cities is discussed in this chapter. It also puts a new tax on the use of ML and deep learning for smart cities and environmental planning with flexible regulations. Cutting trees, support equipment, sensory networks, and Bayesian, neuro-fuzzy and ensembles are the most commonly used ML and DL approaches in smart cities and urban development, according to the study. Due to the intricacy of both the ML and DL approaches, research shows that the use of these algorithms in smart cities faces significant obstacles. Data compatibility and data quality could be a problem when using data.

3.1. Introduction

Urbanization is a key demographic megatrend. According to the United Nations, "the future of the world's population is urban", with urban population growth

Chapter written by Shweta Mayor SABBHARWAL, Manpreet Kaur AIDEN and Sonia CHHABRA.
For a color version of all the figures in this chapter, see www.iste.co.uk/pradhan/cognitivecomputing.zip.

expected to treble by 2050 (Ullah et al. 2020). The author adds that, "cities are the future of the world's population." All of those concerned/involved in developing solutions for sustainable living in urban agglomerations, from academics to visionary enterprises to policymakers all over the world, shake hands in a fast urbanizing world.

The impact of artificial intelligence (AI) on our daily lives is growing by the day. AI is increasingly transforming the nature of our daily jobs, affecting human thought and interaction with the environment in traditional ways. How should the new rules be written to protect current and future generations from the negative effects of AI while maximizing its beneficial effects on humanity? Furthermore, how should AI-assisted rules and laws be designed to assure social and economic progress (O'Dwyer et al. 2019). The authors suggested a smart city crime detection system based on DRL and neural networks to efficiently identify and evaluate any illegal activity.

Machine learning (ML) algorithms are gaining popularity in civil engineering due to their capacity to recognize and categorize patterns in massive datasets (Bhattacharya et al. 2022). The sections that follow provide a categorization of ML algorithms, as well as a study and categorization of ML algorithms that are particularly relevant to smart monitoring applications.

To unearth fresh insights, some ML experts deployed artificial neural networks (ANNs) to examine the SC data. According to the literature, data analytics in SC has been done using shallow ANN and deep learning (DL). DL, on the other hand, has recently piqued academic attention due to its ability to handle massive volumes of data, require less human interaction in data engineering, learn complex structures in huge datasets, and beat shallow ANNs. DL is gaining popularity due to its unique characteristics to cope with large volumes of data without requiring several algorithms for dimensionality reduction, successful work on natural data and the absence of time-consuming human labor required in data engineering (Al-Garadi et al. 2018).

Five advanced ML methodologies have been used so much to deal with the numerous facets of smart cities, according to the report. DL includes ANNs, support vector machines (SVMs), decision trees, and Bayesians, hybrids and neuro-fuzzy ensembles. It has been proven that DL and ML approaches have assisted in solving problems in the fields of energy, healthcare and urban transportation in smart cities (Nosratabadi et al. 2020).

People have been relocating to cities in unprecedented numbers over the last few decades, as cities compress space and speed up time. The year 2008 marked a watershed moment when the urban population overtook that of rural areas for the first time. It is predicted that by 2050, two-thirds of such world population would live in cities. The growing amount of people moving into the area puts enormous strain on municipal infrastructures. Cities have been reliant on technology to maintain life and develop ever more complex technologies and equipment since the dawn of civilization. Cities are like living animals in that they are continually changing.

The smart city is a physical city innovation that combines advanced monitoring with sensor, communication and control technology to give inhabitants real-time, active and intelligent services. Since a smart city should focus on its people's demands, it is critical to infer trends and evaluate citizen behavior in an attempt to improve city services.

A city is indeed a complex system to run, and new ways are needed to make sense of the huge volumes of data it produces. By applying information and communication technologies (ICT) solutions, city administrations can access knowledge hidden in large-scale data to give improved urban governance and management. Better transportation planning, efficient water management, innovative energy efficiency methods, improved trash management and efficient risk management regulations are all possible with these ICT solutions for municipal users.

Furthermore, these ICT solutions can help other essential areas of urban life, including such healthcare system, air quality, pollution and even public security. Large quantities of digital footprints that track individual human activities on both temporal and spatial axes are becoming available as a result of the rapid growth of ICT and pervasive mobile computing. Administrators of smart cities can collect data from a variety of sources. Examples include sensor data from the environment and mobile devices, as well as data from social media (SM).

Data from city-wide sites can be accessed, including power network status, transportation network status, vehicular networks, emergency service provider locations and crowd sizes in various areas throughout the region. Because the gathered data is noisy and redundant, methodical use of data mining (DM) with ML techniques can speed up processing by extracting only important data. ML algorithms have several particular advantages in the extract and release of Big Data services when compared to traditional processing methods. DL, as well as reinforcement learning (RL) approaches, could also accomplish data speed and precision with advanced manipulations.

Hybrid and ensemble approaches are believed to be the most advanced ML and DL methods. Although there have been numerous surveys on the applications of AI, ML and DL techniques in smart cities research, an understanding of the popular methods, categorization of the methods and future trends in the creation of unique methods has yet to be provided (Chakravarthy et al. 2018). As a result, the current study intends to close this gap by presenting the state-of-the-art ML and DL methodologies for smart cities, resulting in a more sustainable approach to urban sustainability. To achieve this, a unique classification is used to identify the most popular ML and DL models, which are then reviewed in separate categories based on the methodologies used (Haase et al. 2018).

Ubiquitous sensing via sensor devices in diverse aspects of network systems is now possible, resulting in intelligent systems in healthcare, transportation, the ecosystem and other relevant branches/networks, due to this rapid progression of sensor technologies, including the IoT and wireless communication (Choudhary et al. 2017). End-user systems are attached thanks to interaction and collaboration among smart systems, culminating in a new integrated unit known as smart cities.

3.2. Basics of machine learning and its implications in smart cities

ML algorithms, on the other hand, must learn from domain experts' experience or expertise. ML algorithms can be classified into several categories depending on the type of learning. Supervised learning, unsupervised learning and RL are the three types of learning (Eremia et al. 2017).

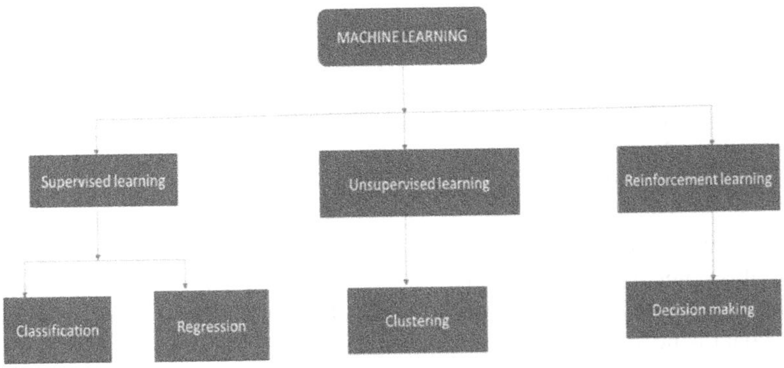

Figure 3.1. *Machine learning algorithms and their categorization*

As shown in Figure 3.1, in supervised learning, ML algorithms use labelEremiaed input–output pairs as training data, and the system learns from the examples provided. In supervised learning, classification and regression issues are the most common. Data is categorized into predetermined categories in classification, while outputs to matching input data are computed in regression

(Choudhary et al. 2017). A major problem in machine learning is unsupervised learning, which is characterized by unlabeled training data. Clustering is the process of grouping data based on similarities. There is no training data in RL. Instead, the system devises a plan to maximize a predetermined total result. The categorization is shown in Figure 3.1. ML algorithms and the subcategories are listed in Figure 3.1.

The process of categorizing a set of data is known as classification. It is possible to use it for both organized and unstructured data. The initial phase in the technique is to predict the class of data points presented. The terms "target", "label" and "categories" are used to describe the classifications. Predictive modeling is the process of calculating the mapping function from discrete input variables to discrete output variables (Chen et al. 2021). The primary goal is to determine which category or class the new information belongs to.

The statistical method of regression is used to determine the relationship between independent variables/features and dependent variables/results. It is used in ML as a method for predictive modeling, in which an algorithm is used to predict continuous outcomes. A key part of every forecasting or predictive model is regression analysis, which is a common approach used in ML-powered predictive analytics. In addition to classification, supervised ML models are frequently used for regression. The usage of tagged input and output training data is required for this method of model training. Because ML regression models must understand the relationship between features and outcomes, appropriately labeled training data is critical.

The most common strategy in unsupervised learning is clustering, which groups data depending on how similar the data points are. Clustering offers a wide range of real-world applications in which it can be applied. The basic premise of clustering is to divide a collection of data into subgroups or clusters with a degree of similarity between observations in the same cluster. It is the use of a person's cognitive ability to distinguish items based on their characteristics. Because there is no external label on the item, it is an unsupervised learning approach. Without any input–output mapping, the machine must learn the characteristics and patterns on its own. The method can derive inferences from the nature of data items and then categorize them into various classes. Because there is no external label on the item, it is an unsupervised learning approach (Garcia-Font et al. 2016). Without any input–output mapping, the machine must learn the characteristics and patterns on its own. The method can derive inferences from the nature of data items and then categorize them into various classes.

ML refers to a machine's capacity to improve through time and mimic human cognitive processes. It is a type of AI that uses computer algorithms. To develop models, these algorithms pick sample data (training data). These models forecast facts from the future and make web-based judgments. It uses human input to learn and make reliable conclusions based on the data. The decision-making process is based on system dynamics and is automated using a variety of technologies, including ML, integrated Big Data tools, decision modeling tools and expert knowledge when needed. Computational statistics is a subfield of ML that focuses on using computers to make judgments and predictions. ML, on the other hand, is not always linked to statistical learning. In the discipline of ML, mathematicians provide theoretical as well as practical applications, as well as the method. DM is also related to this discipline, including unsupervised learning and predictive analysis aimed at exploratory data analysis.

3.3. Basics of deep learning and its implications in smart cities

A complete hierarchy of the deep learning meddlesome and shallow ANN is shown in Figure 3.2. The taxonomy is based on DL and training and shallow ANN, which have been discovered to be used for data analytics in the domain of SC. The concepts of DL for ANN essential concepts on how they operate to achieve their aims are covered in this section, so inquisitive readers can understand how the algorithms work. The DL framework and other narrow ANN given in this section have been determined to be used for data analytics in the SC environment.

Analytics can contribute to advanced findings, a better knowledge of city phenomena, and enable the construction of evidence-based urban plans and innovation in a smart city system. Using a DM method to look for intriguing patterns and connections in developed city, public-service facilities have increasingly become a prominent topic of research. The patterns retrieved can be used to build city layouts or set up new facilities. Advances in large DM technologies can help individuals understand, study and find social and environmental changes, including how people live, behave and show their preferences concerning social trends and public opinions. For data-centric applications in smart cities, DM and ML are critical technologies.

DM is a vast field that encompasses a wide range of algorithms and approaches for extracting information from data, ranging from statistics to ML and information theory. The goal of DM is to create computer programs that can extract hidden, previously undisclosed, and possibly useful facts from data. The procedure must be mechanized, or at the very least semi-automated, as well as the regularities must be useful. Under the features of Big Data, Big DM must expand the full procedure from the front end to the back end. This automatically entails detecting and retrieving implicit hidden rules and knowledge from enormous, heterogeneous data, as well as showing them in an easily accessible format.

ML is indeed the study of how to create computer systems that enhance their performance on certain tasks over time to solve situations where human expertise is lacking or difficult to explain. The algorithm uses this technology to train machines to learn from a previous experience E about a task T and a standard performance P if their performance on T improves with experiences E, calculated by P.

In essence, ML is an AI application that allows computers to learn from data and deliver relevant insights that improve operational efficiency without having to be programmed.

According to Din et al. (2019), ML is divided into four types: supervised learning, unsupervised learning, semi-supervised learning and active learning. Nef et al. (D'Aniello et al. 2018) provide a typical ML pipeline that starts with the raw data to be obtained, grouping to further train the data, and finally classification. The calculated results are then displayed.

Data on both virtual and augmented system entities are consumed by smart city apps. The primary purpose of data collecting is to obtain accurate and complete information. These data, which come from a variety of sources, such as sensors, SM and even manual submissions by users, are unprocessed and loud, and require application processing to be turned into meaningful information. Data preparation is required to harness the data value because entering raw information into the training phase will not generate a reasonable outcome (Shen et al. 2019).

Aside from filthy data, various types of data, including weather conditions, time, etc., are not used effectively for training. The raw data must always be enriched, cleansed, filtered, normalized, verified and arranged in a readable manner to prepare it for processing. Data fusion approaches combine numerous data sources to improve data dependability, complete and extract higher tier information from many data sources.

Several solutions for improving data preparation processes have been presented and used in recent years. In real-world issues, there are hundreds of features to choose from. The primary purpose of information identification is to find a subset of features that are more informative and more predictive of a specific response variable.

A standard feature descriptor is the Bag of Words (BoW). Sajjad et al. suggested a face recognition system based on BoW and the Oriented FAST and Rotated BRIEF (ORB) feature extraction method in their paper.

Principal component analysis is another popular data reduction technique (PCA). The goal of PCA is to reduce attribute overlap. This can be used to determine whether some characteristics are more important than others. The use of dimensionality reduction techniques, such as PCA, minimizes the number of zeros inside the feature matrix and reduces the need for large training datasets. To represent sensor observations, measurements and information and properties of sensing devices, D'Aniello et al. (2018) proposed the semantic sensor network ontology (SSNO) as an ontological system. The SSNO enables us to combine data and information from a sensing device or even a virtual sensor as well as represent them using interoperable statements that can be combined with extra domain knowledge.

3.4. Algorithms of machine learning and deep learning

Sl. no.	Algorithm	Type of the task
1	K-nearest neighbor	Classification problem
2	Naive Bayes	Classification problem
3	Support vector machine	Classification problem
4	Linear regression	Classification/regression problem
5	Random forest	Classification/regression problem
6	K-means	Clustering problem
7	Neural networks	Classification/regression problem
8	Multi-layer perception	Classification/regression problem
9	Bayesian method	Classification problem
10	Radial base function method	Classification problem
11	Model-based method	Clustering problem
12	Hierarchal method	Clustering problem
13	Partition competitive model	Clustering problem

Table 3.1. *Machine learning techniques*

ML algorithms can be used on IoT to enjoy the benefits of cost reductions, increased efficiency and enhanced performance (Liu and Zhang 2021). We have all seen the benefits of ML techniques in the recent period, from streaming movie services that propose titles to watch based on viewing habits to monitoring fraudulent activities based on client spending patterns. It can manage vast amounts of data and derive intriguing patterns or trends, such as anomalies, from them. Machines are required to evaluate data quickly and make choices whenever it reaches a certain level. Table 3.1 lists several ML techniques that help with data processing in industrial IoT devices.

ML algorithms can handle enormous amounts of data and provide features such as mining algorithms, anomaly detection, predictive modeling and optimization, all of which can lead to improved spatial awareness, more efficient, dynamic and effective operations, and adaptive control. Depending on the qualities of the unique application, algorithms perform much better than others depending on the use case requirements. Some ML methods, such as DL, have been designed to improve matching time and accuracy.

3.4.1. *Classification*

The most well-known and often used DM technique is classification. The purpose of classification algorithms is to create functions and models that can be used to determine who among a set of categories (sub-populations) a discovery belongs to, depending on a training dataset containing observations (or instances) with known category membership. Classification is a supervised learning approach (Lima and Teran 2019). The training or construction phase, in which the model learns from a set of labeled samples, and the classification phase, in which the model outputs the label with the highest likelihood for a given sample, are the two fundamental phases of supervised learning. The performance of a classifier is demonstrated to improve as the amount of training data increases (Shen et al. 2019).

3.4.2. *Clustering*

Clustering is one unsupervised approach that classifies a set of data units (clusters) that are not preconceived, unlike classification. Inter-cluster dissimilarity is significant, whereas intra-cluster dissimilarity is modest (according to a set of criteria). Clustering analysis has been widely applied in a variety of applications, including pattern recognition, market analysis and picture segmentation, especially in cases where there is minimal prior information about the data. Clustering algorithms can be classified as hierarchical clustering (HC), partitioned clustering, prototype clustering, density-based grouping, grid-based grouping and so on. Martinez-Espana et al. (2018) used HC methods, which define cluster distance as the largest range between individual components of two clusters. At each phase of the clustering process, the two nearest clusters are united into a new cluster. The two closest clusters are fused into a new cluster at every clustering process. These methods, however, are static, as data objects allocated to one cluster cannot be moved to another. Data items can migrate from one group to another thanks to data migration methods. They can use appropriate models and distance metrics to incorporate knowledge about cluster shape and size.

3.4.3. *K-nearest neighbors*

K-nearest neighbors is indeed a simple regression method that incorporates the average yield of its K-nearest neighbors to estimate the output of new data. The feature set contains the nearest neighbors. This algorithm accumulates the outcomes of the K "closest" cases in the training dataset, wherein K is an essential input to make a forecast. We can use the Euclid or Manhattan distance measurements to calculate the distance between observations. KNN is a type of instance-based learning, often known as passive learning, in which the function is simply investigated locally and all computations are postponed until after classification.

3.4.4. *Naive Bayes*

A Bayesian network (BN) is a compact description of the direct relationships between a collection of statistical variables and a set of nodal probability tables generated in a directed acyclic graph. A BN provides implicit assumptions regarding the dependencies between variables in data modeling, even if two variables are potentially never really and fully independent in the real world. A naive Bayes (NB) classifier is a subset of BN that uses Bayes' theorem in a naive approach by assuming that each predictor is conditionally independent of the category (i.e. attribute) label. As a result, an NB is a straightforward probabilistic classifier based on Bayes' theorem and strong independence assumptions. Brisimi et al. (2018) used the probabilistic ratio test (PRT), an NB classifier that assumes that individual features (elements) in a feature vector x = (x1, …, xn) are unrelated random variables, in their work.

3.4.5. *The support vector machine*

The support vector machine (SVM) is a popular supervised learning model for data classification that has applications in a variety of real-world scenarios, including diagnosis of diseases, event detection, anomaly-based, text categorization, face recognition, power consumption prediction and discovering available parking slots. The SVM training method looks for a feature space separation hyperplane that optimizes the distance between each input piece of data and the hyperplane. Margin is the smallest overall distance. The sample points in real-world data are frequently not linearly separable. As a result, the initial space is mapped into a greater space using a kernel function, where presumably linear segregation can be obtained. Furthermore, even though it overlooks a few misclassified samples, we favor a higher dimensional space that better isolates much of the data. Shen et al. (2019) introduced the secured SVM, which is a secrecy SVM training technique across blockchain-based encrypted IoT data, to close the gap between ideal assumptions and reality restrictions. We could use multi-class SVM to classify the output into additional classes if the method is based on more than two classes. SVM was originally designed to classify the model, but evolved into multi-class classification due to a variety of methodologies. For multi-classification issues, two strategies are commonly used: converting it to several binary classifications and one against one.

3.4.6. *Linear regression*

Linear regression is a numeric variable model in which a single linear function defines the mapping from data to class values. The goal of regression analysis is to represent the relationship between one or more descriptive two or more variables variable. Hashemi chose least squares (LS) among linear regression in his study, which fits a linear dataset by minimizing the total error function. Logistic regression (LogR) is a simple, relatively simple classifier that is used in a wide range of classification applications. The essential concept is that we represent the likelihood function of the responsive class as a likelihood regression with parameters that weight the features f and an offset for each instance. Because it predicts the likelihood of a specimen to the positive class, LogR is widely used in the medical literature. If the data contains a high number of characteristics, we can use the support vector regression, a nonlinear regression technique that supplements the linear regression method. Dynamic time warping is a time-series video, sounds and graphics data sequences algorithm for comparing two provided (time-dependent) patterns that can change in pace (Singh et al. 2017).

3.4.7. *Random forest*

Random forest is a classification and regression ensemble learning model that works by producing a batch of DT at training time. The mean estimate (in regression tasks) or modal of the class (in classification) of a native tree is the output class. Random forests use the simple majority among the outcomes of the developed trees in the aggregate to produce a forecast at a new point. Cross-validation is used to choose the number of trees inside the group. RF performs well on both scaled and unscaled data. It can manage datasets with uneven classes and construct powerful prediction models, effectively avoiding overfitting. The potential to produce high forecast accuracy and the applicability of required capabilities, such as daily power data used by various appliances, make RF an appealing prediction technology. These two features distinguish RF as a desirable model for assessing smart city datasets.

3.4.8. *K-means*

The K-means algorithm is a famous and straightforward partitioning clustering algorithm. The approach is extensible in parallel distributed systems for handling large datasets due to its efficiency. Traditional K-means, on the other hand, are sensitive to the initial cluster center selection and difficult to specify the number of clusters in advance. Aydin et al. (2015) used K-means to cluster two-dimensional GPS location data. Two clustering algorithms were used by Choudhary et al. (2017). Partitioning across medoids (PAM) is a variation of K-means that uses the most representative members in the cluster rather than the centroid as in K-means. The model-based expectation–maximization algorithm, or EM algorithm, is the second approach (EM method). It is a K-means generalization that uses an iterative technique to determine the highest likelihood.

3.4.9. *Artificial neural network*

The artificial neural network (ANN), which is based on supervised learning, is a widely used technology. An ANN is a powerful nonlinear modeling tool that mimics the behavior of biological neurons. Training an ANN entails fine-tuning the network's weights and biases. For the validation data, the goal is to optimize network prediction, which translates into a reduction in the variance among all expected values YK and the intended outputs or targets tk. The NN can learn important statistical information from a reasonable amount of training data to use the backpropagation (BP) method, and the mathematical information gained can describe the function mappings connection of the input–output data model. Multilayer perceptron (MLP), an artificial neural network (NN) with a fully connected topology, is an older ANN architecture. MLP has a good track record and has been frequently used. The radial basis function (RBF) network, used by Olszewski et al. (2018), is a faster-to-train but memory-intensive network for generating a regression model that considers multiple variables. Many novel architectures for ANN have been created recently. ANNs tend to overfit, which means they are trained to suit the noise trend but do not produce the anticipated generalization. By including Bayes' modeling into the regularization scheme, Bayesian regularized ANNs (BRANNs) attempt to avoid the overfitting problem (Li et al. 2019).

The convolutional neural network (CNN) is gaining popularity as a result of its ability to automatically understand underlying patterns from data. The component learning stage and the classifier training stage are the two steps of a CNN's basic structure. A CNN's structure is more sophisticated than a regular NN's (Li et al. 2019). Feedforward neural networks with a recurrent loop are known as recurrent neural networks (RNNs). They are used to solve a wide range of issues involving temporal events that occurred and ordered data. They are regarded as a powerful model for time-series data because they use history. Long short-term memory (LSTM) is indeed a three-layer RNN designed to find a correlation between input and output sequences. Fenza et al. (2019) used LSTM to anticipate energy usage and detect anomalies in a smart energy application. They (Fenza et al. 2019) used a counter-propagation convolutional neural network to identify moving objects with the greatest accuracy (CP-ANN). The CP-ANN seems to have a three-layer design, with an input layer on the first layer, a Kohonen layer on the second layer and a Grossberg layer on the third layer.

While ANNs can extract and model the system's overall behavior, fuzzy logic (FL) modeling can be used for approximation reasoning, modeling qualitative data for inherently occurring uncertainties, and ensuring controllability even in the presence of loud, imprecise data (Hariri et al. 2016). FL also makes it simple to incorporate expert domain expertise into the control system by using linguistic norms that are easily understood by humans, using a well-structured network called the adaptive neuro-fuzzy inference system (ANFIS), which was created by combining ANN and fuzzy systems. They were using the particle swarm optimization (POS) approach to obtain near-optimal control. Evolutionary algorithms (EA) can also be used to dynamically optimize ANN and FL procedures, as well as traditional control methods. EAs are capable of optimizing difficult real-world problems as well as converging on near-optimal outcomes whenever the search space is too huge to be explored exhaustively, as they are inspired by natural selection.

Machine learning refers to a machine's capacity to improve through time and mimic human cognitive processes. It is a type of AI that uses computer algorithms. To develop models, these algorithms pick sample data (training data). These models forecast facts from the future and make web-based judgments. It uses human input to learn and makes reliable conclusions based on the data. The decision-making process is based on system dynamics and is automated using a variety of technologies, including ML, integrated Big Data tools, decision modeling tools and expert knowledge when needed (Nosratabadi et al. 2020).

3.4.10. *Multi-layer perceptron*

The multi-layer perceptron (MLP) is a feed-forward neural network augmentation. The input layer, output layer and hidden layer are the three types of layers represented in Figure 3.2. The input signal to be processed is received by the input layer. The output layer is responsible for tasks such as prediction and categorization. The real computational engine of the MLP is an arbitrary number of hidden layers inserted between the input and output layers. In an MLP, data travels from the input to the output layer in the forward direction, similar to a feed-forward network. Tare is not separable in a linear manner. Pattern categorization, identification, prediction and approximation are some of the MLP's most common applications.

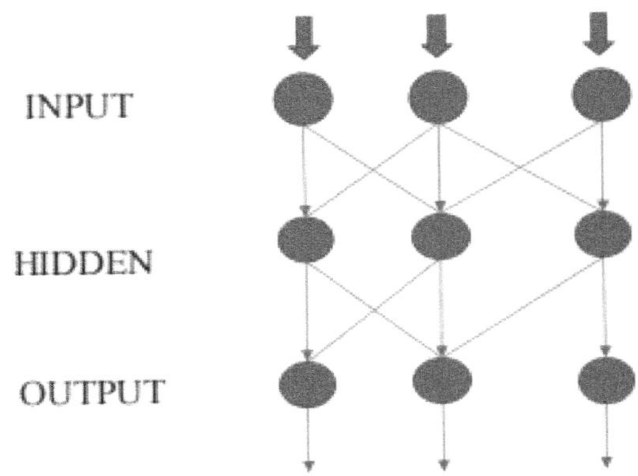

Figure 3.2. *Multi-layer perception*

MLPs can approximate any continuous function rather than only linear functions. They accomplish this by merging several neurons grouped in at least three layers:

– One input layer distributes input characteristics to the first hidden layer.

– Perceptrons in one or more hidden levels. The features dispersed by the input layer are sent into the first hidden layer as inputs. The output of each perceptron from the preceding layer is sent into the other hidden layers.

– One perceptron output layer, which receives as inputs the output of each perceptron from the previously hidden layer.

MLP is frequently used in supervised learning issues, as well as in computational neuroscience and parallel distributed processing research. Speech recognition, picture recognition and machine translation are examples of applications.

3.5. Applications in smart cities using machine learning and deep learning

When a city uses ICT to share data with the public, enhance the quality of government services and increase operational efficiency, it is referred to as a smart city. The main goal of a smart city is to use data analysis and smart technology to improve the city's operations and boost economic growth. The importance of IoT and soft computing technologies in the creation of smart cities is the subject of this chapter. These strategies are used to efficiently construct optimal policies for difficult challenges in smart cities. Various smart city case sectors are investigated, and various ML-based methods are addressed to assist, enhance and fix their challenges. In addition, comparisons are made between the approaches used in existing systems and those used in the proposed system.

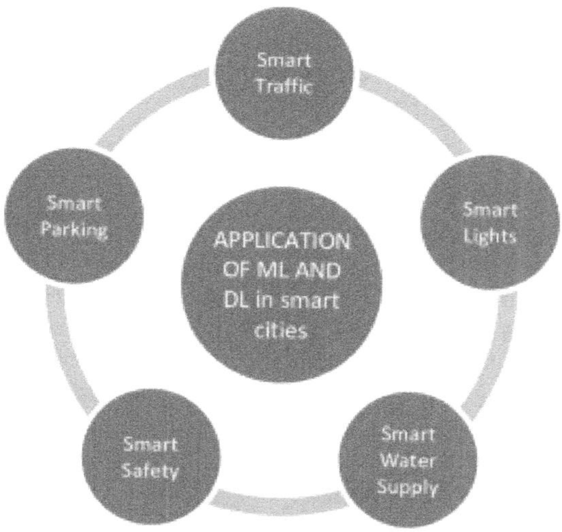

Figure 3.3. *Applications of ML and DL for smart cities*

3.5.1. *Safety of the public*

We can actively use IoT technologies that are focused on giving real-time information via CCTV cameras and sensing instruments to improve public safety in an urban metropolis. The detailed information gathered by these systems aids in the prediction of criminal activity and the implementation of safety measures. The deployment of a gunshot detection system, for example, is the most conspicuous arrangement of safety management. It entails the use of interconnected microphones placed around the city. They regularly gather sound patterns, which are then sent to cloud platforms for processing. ML is then used to filter out the sound of a gunshot. Surprisingly, critical elements like the gun's position can be predicted simply by estimating the sound's speed reaching the listener.

3.5.2. *Intelligent traffic management*

Transportation is one of the most important aspects that can be improved by using smart traffic solutions. The goal is to avoid car coagulation and save citizen's time and fuel. This can be accomplished by placing numerous sensors that can record your vehicle's speed, position and other vital information. AI-assisted traffic sensor systems can use cameras to capture real-time data from cars on the road and send it to a control center, which then collates the data from various sources and changes signal timings to maintain smooth vehicle flow.

The following are some of the helpful systems incorporated in smart traffic management:

– surveillance cams;

– surface sensors for roads;

– platform for traffic management.

All of these technologies work together to collect real-time data, which is subsequently evaluated using ML. As a result, the user receives notifications about traffic congestion, road divergence and other relevant information. Furthermore, historical data can be analyzed using ML to identify peak rush hours.

3.5.3. *Water management strategy*

Water supply and conservation are essential components of sustainable urban life. Establishing a water management system that incorporates gadgets such as smart meters will help track water usage. ML technology can also be used to calculate average consumption for each family, firm or sector. Future consumption statistics can also be predicted using ML algorithms applied to historical data. A smart water management system improves water distribution throughout a city while maintaining water pressure and quality. Several cities around the world have begun to use smart meters to prevent potential leaks in underground water pipelines.

3.5.4. *Smart street lights*

The operation of street lighting can be easily managed with the help of IoT devices. Sensor-equipped street lighting linked to cloud platforms is increasingly adorning smart cities. The sensors help in collecting relevant data such as radiance, public transportation schedules, operating scheduling, etc. When combined with historical data and ML, real-time data is beneficial for analyzing diverse scenarios. As a result, smart lighting systems assist in controlling the brightness and power on/off for streetlights based on traffic volume, time and environmental factors.

3.5.5. *Intelligent parking devices*

We are already aware of the importance of IoT in-car monitoring platforms, thus, its combination with ML can be used to assist smart parking systems. These devices are designed to detect unoccupied parking spaces, particularly in public settings. How does this technology work? The existence of an in-ground vehicle detection sensor, which is embedded into the pavement of various parking places, makes it feasible. They are in charge of gathering data such as the time and duration for which cars used space. The data is then transmitted to the cloud to be analyzed and given to drivers looking for available parking places. ML techniques are also implemented to indicate peak hours achievable with the past trends and real-time data.

3.5.6. *Smart waste and disposal management system*

People who live in cities generate a large quantity of waste, which presents another difficulty for city management in terms of finding the best approach to manage rubbish and keep the environment clean to maintain a high degree of hygiene in society. However, placing AI-enabled sensors on garbage bins can improve waste collection efficiency. Authorities can be notified when the bins are going to be filled, ensuring that operating expenses are reduced by minimizing superfluous collections, giving dynamic collection routes and timetables for waste management optimization.

3.6. Future challenges and research directions

As evidenced by smart city literature, AI-, ML- and DL-based applications have shown promising results. However, academic and industrial experts can concentrate on the following open research challenges that can effectively use AI, ML and DRL to improve the efficiency of smart cities: a substantial set of training data (e.g. vehicle speed, position, vehicle spacing, driver behavior, UAV height, relay BS, etc.) is needed to properly train the ML and DRL protocols for more accurate and precise decision-making procedures. Co-optimization of UAV onboard capabilities (e.g. caching, navigation, etc.) (resources for computation, processing, sensing and communication) and its trajectory can be considerably improved by using ML techniques. Standardization of Big Data creation in SGs, communication protocols used during device interoperability and selection of the most efficient AI, ML and DRL techniques can boost SG performance to near-optimal levels.

5G technology is scheduled to be adopted in 2020, necessitating the standardization of SG communication infrastructure to ensure effective compatibility between existing SGs and future 5G technology. Any SG or electric company's primary priority is the optimization of power-down scenarios. The lag in communication to build an effective system, assessment analysis is an essential network. The use of ML and DL techniques can help develop strategies for switching between 5G and 4G networks while ensuring that power is delivered in a consistent manner supply. Another fundamental difficulty with the SC is the ever-changing nature of technical progress: as technology advances, so does the notion of the SC. The further evolution of the SC may represent a challenge to DL models, as it may present difficulties in managing the novel notion of SC data analytics from future generations of SC.

Due to the vast number of overt and covert dimension factors and criteria, making judgments in smart cities is difficult. In this chapter, we will look at one of the most important areas of smart cities, smart mobility, and how it influences smart city decision-making. Cognitive decision-making control systems in sustainable mobility have a lot of benefits, including efficiency improvements, traffic relaying information (Kothai et al. 2021) and, most crucially, reduced air pollution by providing real-time, actionable information and critically established knowledge. With such a varied choice of smart devices and systems, it is difficult to pick the best option at the right moment in smart mobility. If our data is not captured regularly, we will not be able to make good decisions. As a result, owing to resource scarcity, decision support system training remains difficult.

3.7. Conclusion

We looked at current smart city research trends and developments, as well as the work done by academics and businesses on a variety of challenging topics and applications. A basic understanding of AI, ML and DL approaches has been created. We discussed the latest AI, ML and DRL applications in smart city governance, as well as the need for AI-assisted and AI-compatible new rules, energy-efficient ITS, SGs, cybersecurity and UAV-assisted 5G and B5G communications. We briefly discussed the expanding relevance of the aforementioned approaches in smart healthcare, ranging from efficient diagnosis to health recovery, the security of health-oriented IoT devices and the potential function of these technologies in the future.

The processes investigated in this study are ANNs, SVM, ensembles (probabilistic theorems, hybrids, and neuro-fuzzy), and DL, which are used to provide various approaches for the energy sector, making it the area that has most invested ML and DL strategies in the development of smart cities. Other smart cities realms that have succeeded in getting the most attention of researchers in the standard disciplines of ML and DL methods and smart cities in which at least three distinct ML and DL strategies are used to answer their research questions include energy, health, urban transportation and smart city management and monitoring.

3.8. References

Al-Garadi, M.A., Mohamed, A., Al-Ali, A., Du, X., Guizani, M. (2018). A survey of the machine and deep learning methods for internet of things (IoT) security. arXiv preprint arXiv:1807.11023.

AlZoman, R.M. and Alenazi, M.J.F. (2021). A comparative study of traffic classification techniques for smart city networks. *Sensors*, 21(14), 4677. doi: 10.3390/s21144677.

Aydin, G., Hallac, I.R., Karakus, B. (2015). Architecture and implementation of a scalable sensor data storage and analysis system using cloud computing and big data technologies. *Journal of Sensors*, 834217.

Bhattacharya, S., Somayaji, S.R.K., Gadekallu, T.R., Alazab, M., Maddikunta, P.K.R. (2022). A review on deep learning for future smart cities. *Internet Technology Letters*, 5(1). doi: 10.1002/itl2.187.

Brisimi, T.S., Xu, T., Wang, T., Dai, W., Adams, W.G., Paschalidis, I.C. (2018). Predicting chronic disease hospitalizations from electronic health records: An interpretable classification approach. *Proceedings of the IEEE*, 106, 690–707.

Chakravarthy, S., Schmitt, S., Yang, L. (2018). Intelligent crime anomaly detection in smart cities using deep learning. In *2018 IEEE 4th International Conference on Collaboration and Internet Computing*, 399–404.

Chen, Q., Wang, W., Wu, F., De, S., Wang, R., Zhang, B., Huang, X. (2019). A survey on an emerging area: Deep learning for smart city-data. *IEEE Transactions on Emerging Topics in Computational Intelligence*, 3(5), 392–410.

Chen, D., Wawrzynski, P., Lv, Z. (2021). Cyber security in smart cities: A review of deep learning-based applications and case studies. *Sustainable Cities and Society*, 66, 102655.

Choudhary, S.K., Sathe, R.B., Kachare, A.E. (2017) Smart cities based on Internet of Things (IoT). *International Journal of Engineering Trends and Technology – IJETT*, 48(8), 434–439.

D'Aniello, G., Gaeta, M., Orciuoli, F. (2018). An approach based on semantic stream reasoning to support decision processes in smart cities. *Telematics and Informatics*, 35, 68–81.

Din, I.U., Guizani, M., Rodrigues, J., Hassan, S., Korotaev, V. (2019). Machine learning in the internet of things: Designed techniques for smart cities. *Future Generation Computer Systems*, 100, 826–843.

Eremia, M., Toma, L., Sanduleac, M. (2017). The smart city concept in the 21st century. *Procedia Engineering*, 181, 15–21.

Fenza, G., Gallo, M., Loia, V. (2019). Drift-aware methodology for anomaly detection in smart grid. *IEEE Access*, 7, 9645–9657.

Garcia-Font, V., Garrigues, C., Rifa-Pous, H. (2016). A comparative study of anomaly detection techniques for smart citywireless sensor networks. *Sensors*, 16, 868. doi: 10.3390/s16060868.

Golubchikov, O. and Thornbush, M. (2020). Artificial intelligence and robotics in smart city strategies and planned smart development. *Smart Cities*, 3(4), 1133–1144. doi: 10.3390/smartcities3040056.

Elmqvist, T. (ed.) (2018). *The Urban Planet: Knowledge Towards Sustainable Cities*. Cambridge University Press, Cambridge.

Hariri, R., Fredericks, E.M., Bowers, K.M. (2016). Uncertainty in big data analytics: Survey, opportunities, and challenges. *Journal of Big Data*, 6, 1–16.

Hurbean, L., Danaiata, D., Militaru, F., Dodea, A.M., Negovan, A.M. (2021). Open data-based machine learning applications in smart cities: A systematic literature review. *Electronics*, 10(23), 2997. doi: 10.3390/electronics10232997.

Kothai, G., Poovammal, E., Dhiman, G., Ramana, K., Sharma, A., AlZain, M.A., Gaba, G.S., Masud, M. (2021). A new hybrid deep learning algorithm for prediction of wide traffic congestion in smart cities. *Wireless Communications and Mobile Computing*, 1–13.

Li, D., Deng, L., Gupta, B.B., Wang, H., Choi, C. (2019). A novel CNN based security guaranteed image watermarking generation scenario for smart city applications. *Information Science*, 479, 432–447.

Li, X., Liu, H., Wang, W., Zheng, Y., Lv, H., Lv, Z. (2022). Big data analysis of the Internet of Things in the digital twins of smart city based on deep learning. *Future Generation Computer Systems*, 128, 167–177.

Lima, S. and Teran, L. (2019). Cognitive smart cities and deep learning: A classification framework. *2019 Sixth International Conference on EDemocracy & EGovernment (ICEDEG)*, 180–187. doi: 10.1109/ICEDEG.2019.8734346.

Liu, L. and Zhang, Y. (2021). Smart environment design planning for the smart city is based on deep learning. *Sustainable Energy Technologies and Assessments*, 47, 101425.

Luckey, D., Fritz, H., Legatiuk, D., Dragos, K., Smarsly, K. (2021). Artificial intelligence techniques for smart city applications. *The International ICCCBE and CIB W78 Joint Conference on Computing in Civil and Building Engineering 2020*, Sao Paolo, 3–15.

Martinez-Espana, R., Bueno-Crespo, A., Timon, I., Soto, J., Munoz, A., Cecilia, J.M. (2018). Air-pollution prediction in smart citiesthrough machine learning methods: A case study in Murcia, Spain. *Journal of Universal Computer Science*, 24, 261–276.

Mohapatra, B.N. and Panda, P.P. (2019). Machine learning applications to smart city. *ACCENTS Transactions on Image Processing and Computer Vision*, 5(14), 1–6. doi: 10.19101/TIPCV.2018.412004.

Nosratabadi, S., Mosavi, A., Keivani, R., Ardabili, S., Aram, F. (2020). State of the art survey of deep learning and machine learning models for smart cities and urban sustainability. *International Conference on Global Research and Education*, 228–238. doi: 10.48550/arXiv.2010.02670.

O'Dwyer, E., Pan, I., Acha, S., Shah, N. (2019). Smart energy systems for sustainable smart cities: Current developments, trends, and future directions. *Applied Energy*, 237, 581–597.

Oladipo, I.D., AbdulRaheem, M., Bamidele, A.J., Bhoi, A.K., Adeniyi, E., Abiodun, M. (2022). Machine learning and deep learning algorithms for smart cities: A start-of-the-art review. *IoT and IoE Driven Smart Cities*, 143–162.

Olszewski, R., Palka, P., Turek, A. (2018). Solving "Smart City" transport problems by designing carpooling gamification schemes with multi-agent systems: The case of the so-called "Mordor of Warsaw". *Sensors*, 18, 141.

Shen, M., Tang, X., Zhu, L., Du, X., Guizani, M. (2019). Privacy-preserving support vector machine training over blockchain-based encrypted IoT data in smart cities. *IEEE Internet of Things Journal*, 6, 7702–7712.

Singh, G., Bansal, D., Sofat, S. (2017). A smartphone based technique to monitor driving behavior using DTW and crowdsensing. *Pervasive and Mobile Computing Journal*, 40, 56–70.

Ullah, Z., Al-Turjman, F., Mostarda, L., Gagliardi, R. (2020). Applications of artificial intelligence and machine learning in smart cities. *Computer Communications*, 154, 313–323.

Wang, S.J. and Moriarty, P. (eds) (2018). Urban health and well-being challenges. In *Big Data for Urban Sustainability*. Springer, Cham.

4

An Intelligent Healthcare System Based on Machine Learning Models for Accurate Detection of Heart Disease

Heart disease (HD) is the major cause of death in the recent era. Due to unhealthy lifestyles, the death rate has increased rapidly in recent years due to HD. If the disease is detected early, many people's lives could be saved. The main objective of this study is to develop an automatic HD detection system using machine learning (ML) models and to compare their performance in terms of training as well as testing accuracy, F1-score and AUC. Five ML models, namely support vector machine (SVM), random forest (RF), multilayer perceptron (MLP), stochastic gradient descent (SGD) and naive Bayes (NB), were used in this study and obtained an accuracy of 88.59, an F1-score of 90.58 and an AUC of 0.92 using the SVM model. Similarly, an accuracy of 86.41, an F1-score of 88.58 and an AUC of 0.93 were obtained using the RF model. Using an MLP classifier, an accuracy of 84.78, an F1-score of 87.27 and an AUC of 0.92 were obtained. Using an SGD model, an accuracy of 82.61, an F1-score of 85.31 and an AUC of 0.89 were obtained for HD detection. Using the NB model, we obtained an accuracy of 83.77, an F1-score of 84 and an AUC of 0.91. The dataset used for the experimental work was downloaded from the UCI repository site and contains 918 samples. The ML-based forecasting model in this study is effective for the early diagnosis of HD. This work provides encouraging findings that point to the potential usefulness of ML-based computer-aided diagnostic systems as diagnostic tools for identifying previously undetected heart illnesses in primary healthcare facilities around the world.

Chapter written by Madhumita PAL, Smita PARIJA, Ganapati PANDA and Ranjan K. MOHAPATRA.

For a color version of all the figures in this chapter, see www.iste.co.uk/pradhan/cognitivecomputing.zip.

4.1. Introduction

Cardiovascular diseases (CVDs) are the most common cause of death worldwide. According to estimates, 17.9 million deaths worldwide in 2019 were attributable to CVDs, or 32% of all fatalities, and it is expected that this number would continue to rise in the years to come. Heart attack and stroke deaths accounted for 85% of these fatalities. The majority of CVD fatalities occur in low- and middle-income nations. In 2019, noncommunicable illnesses caused 17 million premature deaths (before the age of 70), and 38% of those fatalities were attributable to CVD (see: https://www.who.int/news-room/fact sheets/detail/cardio vascular-diseases-(cvds)). By addressing behavioral risk factors such as tobacco use, unhealthy eating and obesity, inactivity and problematic alcohol consumption, the majority of cardiovascular illnesses can be avoided.

Early detection of CVD is crucial in order to start treatment with counseling and medication. While early detection of heart-related illnesses is beneficial, it is challenging because chest pain symptoms vary in their severity. Although electrocardiograms are a promising technology, they are not sensitive enough to detect minute variations in a heartbeat. A variety of disorders that affect the heart are referred to as heart diseases. Heart conditions comprise diseases of the blood vessels, such as coronary artery disease, abnormal heartbeats (arrhythmias), heart problems by birth (congenital heart defects) and muscular disease of the heart (see: https://www.cdc.gov/heartdisease/about.html). The body's cardiovascular system, which also encompasses the lungs, is composed mostly of the heart, a type of muscular organ that controls blood flows into the body. The heart muscle is also made up of a network of blood vessels, such as capillaries, arteries and veins. These blood vessels distribute blood throughout the body. Cardiovascular disorders, often known as heart disorders, are characterized by deviations from the heart's normal blood flow. The leading causes of death worldwide are heart disorders. According to a survey conducted by the World Health Organization (WHO), heart attacks and strokes are responsible for 17.5 million deaths worldwide. Most deaths from heart events – 75% of them – occur in middle- and low-income nations. Heart disease can be treated easily if it is detected at an early stage. Different noninvasive tests such as echocardiogram, MRI test, CT scan test, and electrocardiogram and invasive tests such as angiography and electrophysiology are recommended by doctors to examine the heart condition. But all of these tests are time-consuming, expensive and sometimes error-prone. To overcome this problem, an automatic heart disease detection system is developed using ML models for early detection of the disease.

Recently, due to Covid-19 pandemic, millions of people also suffered from heart disease due to the use of steroids in the treatment (Mohapatra et al. 2021, 2022; Pal et al. 2022a, 2022b). Post-Covid-19 also had a major impact on the human heart condition, which can lead to death in many people. So, early detection of heart disease is also an important challenge for the doctors. The main objective of the study is to develop an automatic heart disease detection system for the early prediction of the disease using python open-source software based on ML models.

The rest of this chapter is organized as follows: section 4.2 presents the work done by the researchers for heart disease prediction using ML methods. Section 4.3 presents the methods used for HD detection. The simulation result part is explained in section 4.4. The conclusion of the article is described in section 4.5.

4.2. Literature survey

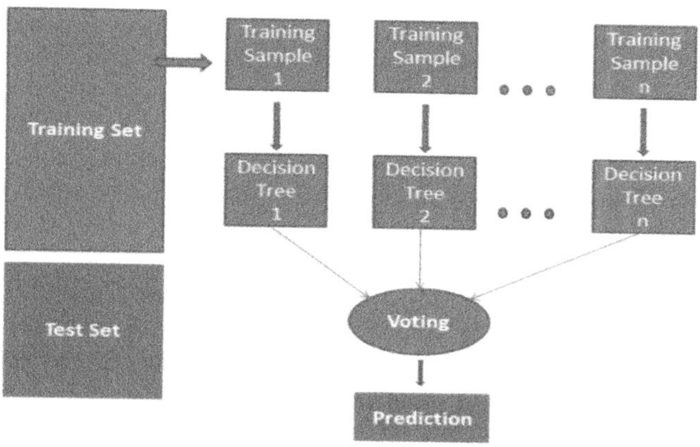

Figure 4.1. *HD detection using random forest (see: https://www.who.int/news-room/fact sheets/detail/cardiovascular-diseases-(cvds))*

The system for detecting cardiac illness using artificial intelligence (AI) and machine learning (ML) algorithms was proposed by Chang et al. (2022), as shown in Figure 4.1. They have demonstrated how AI can be used to forecast if someone is likely to suffer from a cardiac disease. They have created a python-based application for healthcare research in this study since it is more dependable and aids in tracking and establishing various kinds of health monitoring applications. They have demonstrated categorical variable manipulation and the conversion of categorical columns in data processing and outlined the key stages of application development, including the gathering of databases, applying logistic regression and assessing the features of the dataset. They have implemented a RF classifier method with an 83%

accuracy rate, which requires data analysis. According to Guleria and Sood's (2020) description, doctors and institutions can offer patients better and improved outcomes through scalable and dynamic apps by implementing python programming in the healthcare sectors, particularly for identifying cardiac problems.

Heart disease is a fatal human disease, and needs early and on-time diagnosis. In this context, Muhammad et al. (2020) reported an intelligent computational predictive system as effectual for the heart disease diagnosis. The authors investigated various ML algorithms in the study. Several performance metrics are used to observe the effectiveness of this developed model. The chi-square and P-value are also computed for the ET classifier. This developed model will be helpful to diagnose the heart disease effectively by the physician in the early stage. New opportunities are emerging to build AI tools with the advent of Big Data and ML for the diagnosis of CVD. In this context, Martin-Isla et al. (2020) discussed various ML methods that can be helpful in enabling more automated, precise and early diagnosis of CVD. Nagavelli et al. (2022) compared four ML models in terms of performance parameters (accuracy, precision, f1-measure and recall), which will be helpful for the early diagnosis of heart problems in patients. This study uses XG Boost as a hope to improve the accuracy of heart disease diagnosis. Dev et al. (2022) analyzed various factors for effective stroke prediction by using various statistical techniques and principal component analysis. The study concluded that age, average glucose level, heart disease and hypertension are important factors for detecting stroke. With these attributes, a perceptron neural network provides the highest accuracy rate, which will be helpful for better patient management. Pal et al. (2021) predicted CVD using MLP and obtained an accuracy and AUC of 82.47% and 86.41% respectively.

4.3. Features of the dataset

The dataset used for the experimental work was accessed from the University of California Irvine repository site (see: https://archive.ics.uci.edu/ml/datasets/heart+disease). The dataset contains 918 samples and 11 features. The features of the dataset are explained in Table 4.1. Python open-source software is used for the experimental work. The simulation work was performed using jupyter notebook environment. Pandas, Num Py, sklearn, sea born and mat plot lib packages were used for the simulation work.

Sl no.	Features	Description
1.	Age	Age of the patient in years:
2.	Sex	Gender of the patient: Male = 0 Female = 1
3.	Cp	Chest pain types: 0: typical angina 1: atypical angina 2: non-anginal pain 3: asymptomatic (nominal)
4.	trestbps	Patient blood pressure at rest condition
5.	Cholesterol	Serum cholesterol level of the patient in mm/dl
6.	fbs	Fasting blood sugar 1: fbs > 120 0: otherwise
7.	restecg	Resting electrocardiogram results
9.	MaxHR	Maximum heart rate achieved (between 60 and 202)
10.	Exercise angina	Exercise-induced angina Y: yes N: no
11.	oldpeak	Exercise-induced ST depression
12.	ST_slope	ST segment measured in terms of slope during exercise
13.	Heart disease	1: yes 0: no

Table 4.1. *Features of the dataset used for the experimental work*

The heart disease dataset contains 11 features and one target feature. Among these 12 features, seven are numerical features, namely "Age", "Resting BP", "Cholesterol", "Fasting BS", "Max HR", "Old peak", "Heart disease" and five are categorical features such as "Sex" (Figure 4.2), "Chest pain type" (Figure 4.3), "Resting ECG" (Figure 4.4), "Exercise angina" (Figure 4.5) and "ST_slope" (Figure 4.6).

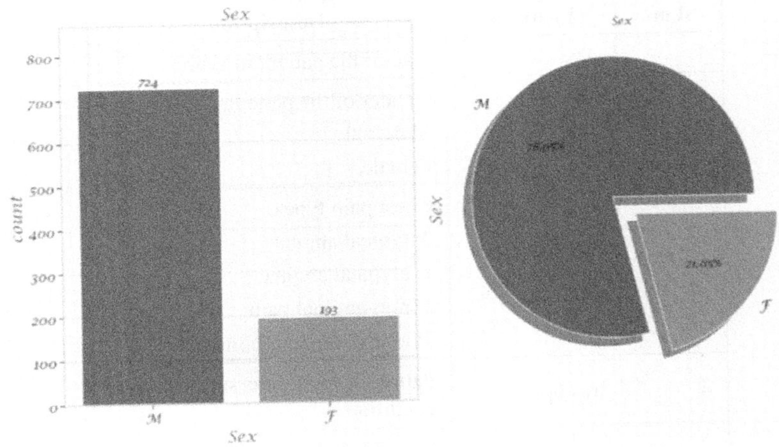

Figure 4.2. *Number of male and female patients suffering from heart disease*

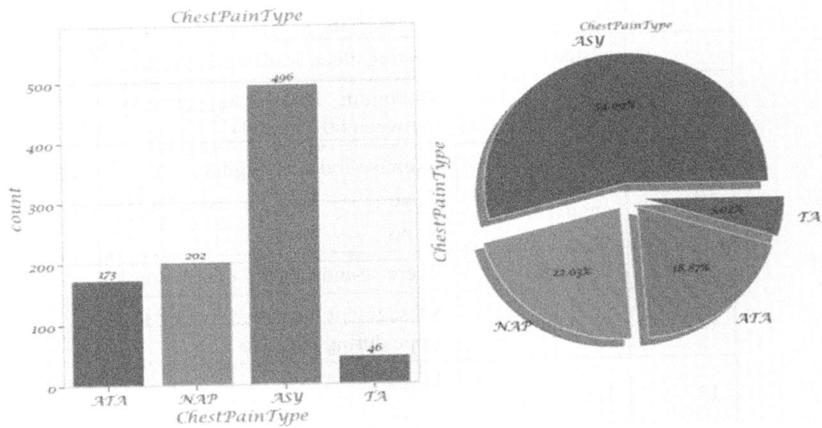

Figure 4.3. *Count plot for the number of patients suffering from different types of chest pain*

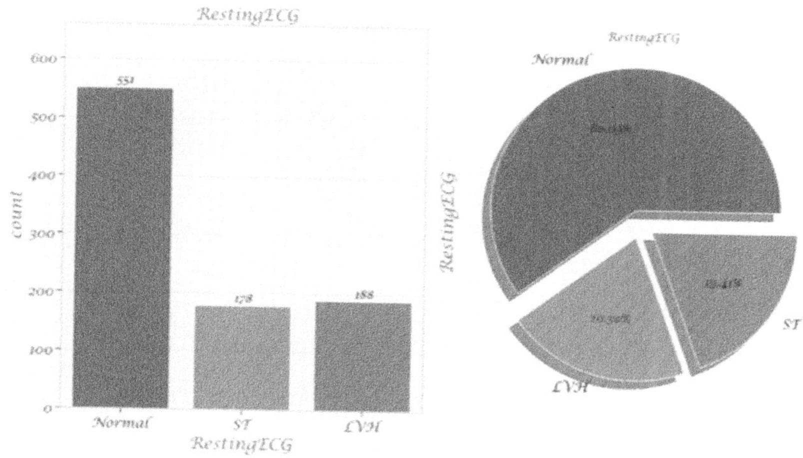

Figure 4.4. *Number of patients with normal ECG signals and abnormal ECG signals*

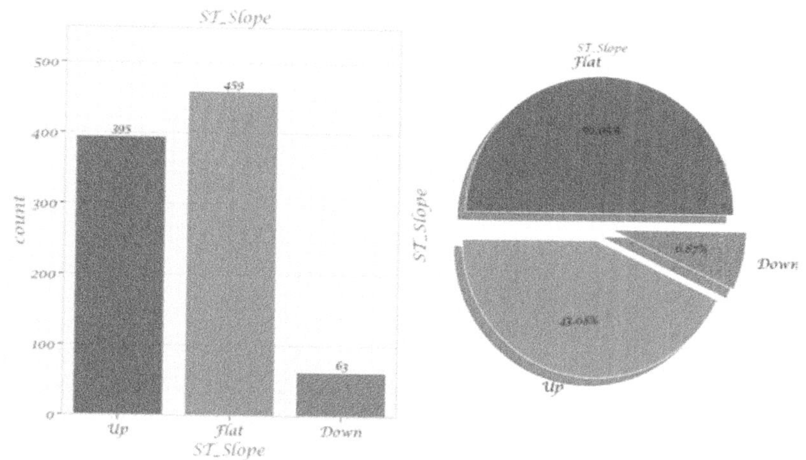

Figure 4.5. *Count plot for the number of patients with different types of ST_slope*

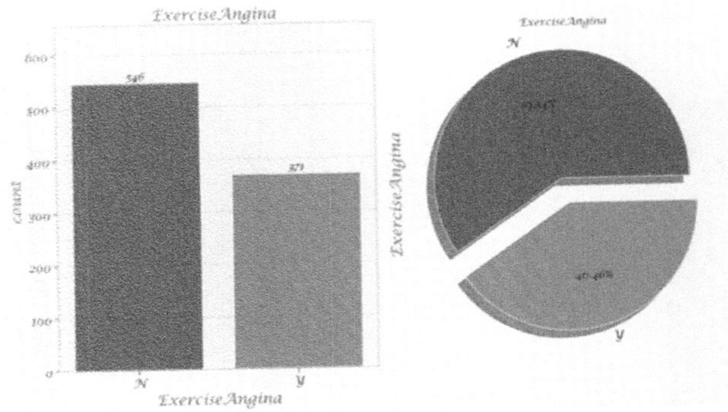

Figure 4.6. *Number of patients suffering from angina problem*

Machine learning (ML) is a subset of AI that is infiltrating scientific study in ever-increasing ways.

4.4. Proposed system

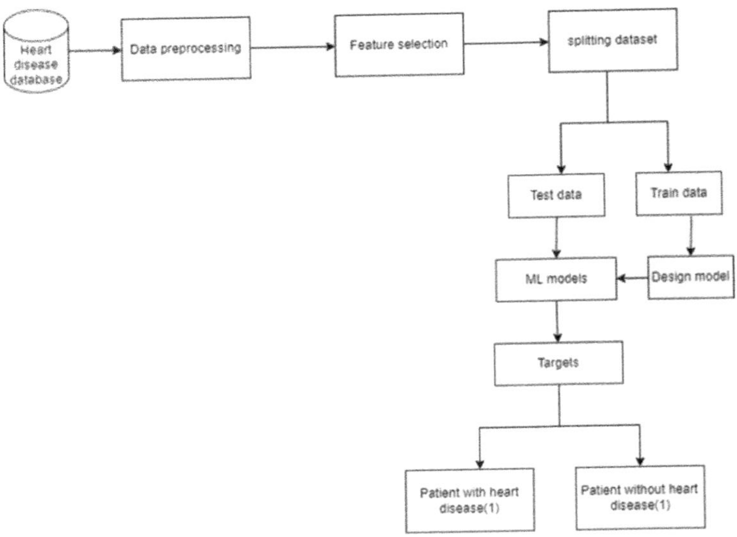

Figure 4.7. *Schematic block diagram for HD detection*

As shown in Figure 4.2, data was preprocessed in the data preprocessing phase, and during this phase, missing values and null values were removed from the dataset. Features are selected during the feature selection phase. Overall, 80% of the data was used for training the model, and 20% of the data was used for testing. Five ML models, namely SVM, RF, SGD, MLP and NB classifiers, are implemented on the dataset for classifying a normal patient from a heart disease patient.

4.5. ML models used for the experimental work

ML is crucial in determining whether or not heart arrhythmia, motor problems, heart illnesses and other conditions exist. It was anticipated that it would give doctors important new information that would enable them to customize each patient's diagnosis and care.

4.5.1. *Support vector machines (SVM)*

One of the most well-liked algorithms for supervised learning is called the support vector machine (SVM), and it is used to solve both classification and regression issues. However, it is mainly used in machine learning classification issues. The objective of the SVM algorithm is to establish the best decision boundary or line that can divide n-dimensional space into classes so that subsequent data points can be quickly assigned to the appropriate category. The term "hyperplane" refers to this optimal decision boundary. This is one of the efficient supervised algorithms used for solving classification problems along with regression problems (Zahariev et al. 2020). This model divides positive classes and negative classes. Input to this model is given as Train data (Wang and Liang 2018). The model performance is measured through test data. SVM selects the extreme vectors and points that aid in the creation of the hyperplane. Support vectors, which are used to represent these extreme instances, form the basis for the SVM method.

4.5.2. *Random forest (RF)*

A large number of decision trees are built during the training phase of the random forests (RF) or random decision forests ensemble learning approach, which is used for classification, regression and other tasks. The class that the majority of the trees chose is the output of the RF for classification problems. The mean or average prediction of each individual tree is returned for regression tasks. The tendency of decision trees to overfit their training set is corrected by random decision forests. Although they frequently outperform decision trees, gradient boosted trees are more accurate than random forests. This algorithm proves that the data is reliable and highly accurate. The number of participatory decision trees that can be used in the process is also supported by this algorithm. It does not cause problems with overfitting. This is because it eliminates prejudice by taking the average of all predictions into account. This RF approach is helpful for both classification and regression problems (Noshad et al. 2019). This model is an ensemble learning technique used for handling classification and regression problem. It is the combination of many decision trees. The accuracy of the model is improved by using majority voting, bootstrap as well as bagging technique. As the name suggests, in this model, samples are selected randomly and by using the bagging and boosting technique, the model accuracy can be improved. In this algorithm, entropy is used for separating the classes. The parameters XTest and YTest are used in the method score to determine the score of this model (Mehrang et al. 2018).

The entropy criterion is represented by Entropy=$-\sum$Pi .log2(Pi) [4.1]

4.5.3. *Stochastic gradient descent (SGD) method*

In ML applications, SGD is a common optimization approach used to identify the model parameters that best match the expected and observed outputs. It is an imperfect yet effective strategy. SGD is a system or process associated with a random probability and is referred to as stochastic. As a result, for each iteration of SGD, a small number of samples are chosen at random rather than the entire dataset. In SGD, each iteration is carried out with just one sample, or a batch size of one. For the iteration, the sample is chosen and randomly shuffled. The learning rate hyperparameters, which control the step size, are a crucial gradient descent (GD) parameter. It will take a very long time for the algorithm to converge if the learning rate is too low, and it may cause us to jump the optimal value if it is too high.

SGD equation is given as follows:

$$\theta_i = \theta_i - \eta(\hat{y}_i - y_i)x_i \quad [4.2]$$

where:

η represents the learning parameter;

xi represents the input vectors;

y_i represents the output vector;

$\hat{y}_i$ represents the predicted output.

This algorithm works as follows:

1) For each parameter or feature, the slope of the goal function, i.e. the function's gradient, is found.

2) A random starting point for each parameter has been chosen.

3) The parameter values are updated to update the gradient function.

4) Step sizes should be determined using the formula: step size = gradient * learning rate.

5) The new parameters are created by subtracting the previous parameters by the step size.

6) When the gradient is nearly zero, steps 3–5 are repeated.

4.5.4. *Multilayer perceptron (MLP)*

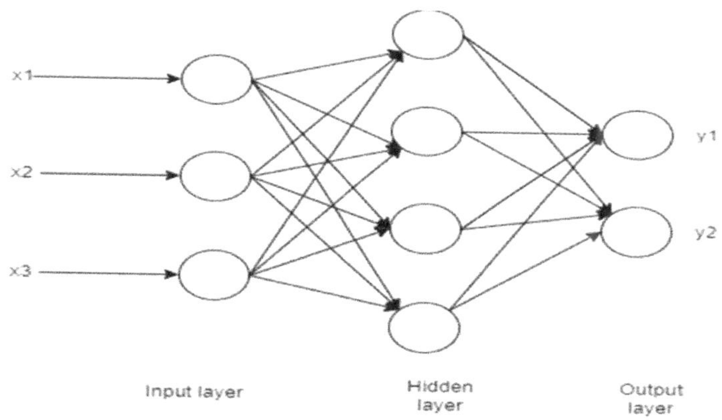

Figure 4.8. *Architecture of MLP diagram*

It is a simple feed-forward supervised ML algorithm. It consists of three layers: the input layer, the hidden layer and the output layer (Figure 4.8). Information passes from the input layer to the output layer through the hidden layer in the forwarding direction. Each layer consists of nodes that depend upon the information bits passed through the network. Errors of information bits are corrected using the back-propagation training algorithm. All nodes except for the input node use the nonlinear activation function such as sigmoid and Tanh. The input layer is where the input features (x1, x2, x3) for processing are received. The output layer (y1,y2) completes the necessary task, such as classification and prediction. Data flows from the input to the output layer of an MLP in the forward direction, much like a feed-forward network. The neurons of the MLP are trained with the help of the back-propagation learning algorithm.

The input features are given to a function that receives them and computes the weighted sum of the input features:

$$v(x) = \sum_{j=1}^{n} \omega_j x_j \qquad [4.3]$$

The output of the input perceptron is passed by an activation function f, which receives the outcome of this calculation. The activation function of the original perceptron is a step function:

$$y = f(v(x))=\{1,\text{if}\, v(x)>\theta,\ 0 \text{ otherwise} \qquad [4.4]$$

$$\theta = \text{Threshold. parameter}$$

4.5.5. *Naive Bayes (NB)*

This Bayes theorem-based (equation [4.5]) ML model is used for disease classification, text separation and classification of spam mails. NB is a simple and easy-to-implement algorithm, and due to its simplicity, the algorithm could outperform a more complex model if the size of the dataset is not large enough. In the classification case, it is used for text classification. Keywords can be present or absent in the case of text classification. NB can be used for disease classification

$$P\left(\frac{A}{B}\right)=\frac{P\left(\frac{B}{A}\right)P(A)}{P(B)} \qquad [4.5]$$

where P(A|B) is the posterior probability, P(B|A) is the likelihood probability, P(A) is the prior probability and P(B) is the marginal probability.

4.6. Performance parameters of ML models

4.6.1. *Confusion matrix*

It is a performance matrix that evaluates the performance of ML models.

True positive (TP): both the predicted value and the output value are positive. If it is predicted that a person is suffering from HD, and the doctor confirmed that the person is actually suffering from HD is an example of a true positive case. True negative (TN): correctly predicted a negative outcome. You correctly anticipated that a person is not suffering from HD, and that is the case. False positive (FP: type 1 error): if the predicted value is positive and the actual value is negative. For example, even though a person has HD, it is actually not the case. False negative (FN: type 2 error): prediction of a negative result was incorrect. Despite the correct prediction, the person has HD.

4.6.2. *Accuracy*

Accuracy defines how accurately ML models can classify a normal patient from a heart disease patient. The formula for accuracy calculation is given as follows:

$$\text{Accuracy} = \frac{\text{TP+TN}}{\text{TP+FP+TN+FN}} \qquad [4.6]$$

4.6.3. *F1-score*

It is the arithmetic mean of precision and recall. The formula for the F1-score is given as follows:

$$\text{F1-Score} = (2\times \frac{\text{TP}}{\text{TP+FP}} \times \frac{\text{TP}}{\text{TP+FN}}) \div (\frac{\text{TP}}{\text{TP+FP}} + \frac{\text{TP}}{\text{TP+FN}}) \qquad [4.7]$$

4.6.4. *AUC*

It is used to assess and compare the effectiveness of binary classification models. It evaluates the classification model's predictive capacity and how well the model can distinguish (separate) events and nonevents. It is a plot drawn between TPR against FPR. The formula for TPR and FPR is given as follows:

$$\text{TPR (True positive rate), TPR.} = \frac{\text{TP}}{\text{TP+FN}} \qquad [4.8]$$

$$\text{FPR} = \frac{\text{FP.}}{\text{TN+FP}} \qquad [4.9]$$

4.7. Result and analysis

The dataset used for the experimental work was accessed from the UCI repository site. Different ML models are implemented on the heart disease dataset, and their performance is measured in terms of accuracy, AUC and F1-score. The obtained confusion matrices of different ML models are shown in Figure 4.9. Different parameter values of the confusion matrix are shown in Table 4.2.

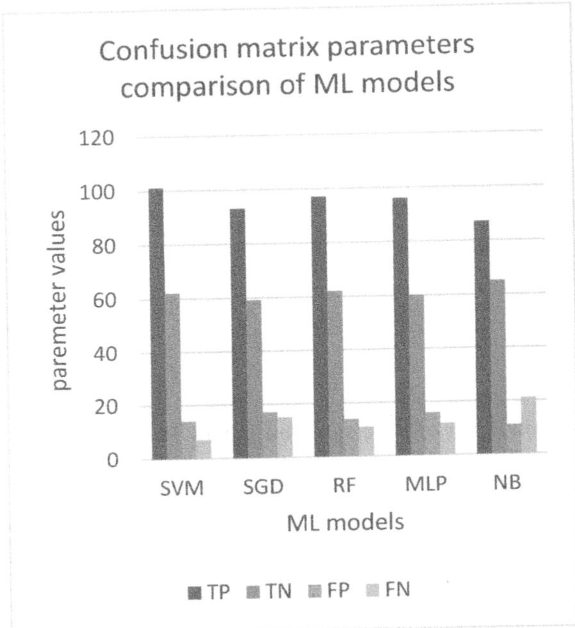

Figure 4.9. *Confusion matrix parameter comparison of ML models*

ML models	TP	TN	FP	FN
SVM	101	62	14	7
SGD	93	59	17	15
RF	97	62	14	11
MLP	96	60	16	12
NB	87	65	11	21

Table 4.2. *Values of confusion matrix parameters of ML models*

The performance of each of these models is measured in terms of accuracy, F1-score and AUC parameters, and their values are given in Table 4.3.

ML models	Training accuracy	Model accuracy	F1-score	AUC
SVM	87.31	88.59	90.58	0.92
RF	100	84.78	87.39	0.92
SGD	84.17	83.70	87.07	0.89
MLP	88.40	85.33	87.89	0.92
NB	83.77	83.61	84.47	0.91

Table 4.3. *Values of ML model performance parameters*

ML model testing accuracy has been compared, as shown in Figure 4.10. From the figure, it can be seen that the SVM model has the highest testing accuracy of 88.59, followed by the MLP (85.33), RF (84.78), SGD (83.70) and NB (83.61) models. The ROC–AUC curve of the SVM model is shown in Figure 4.11.

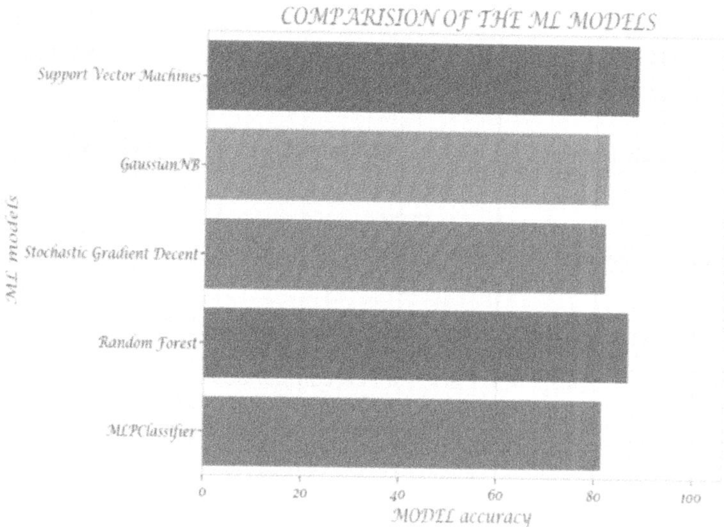

Figure 4.10. *Testing accuracy comparison of ML models*

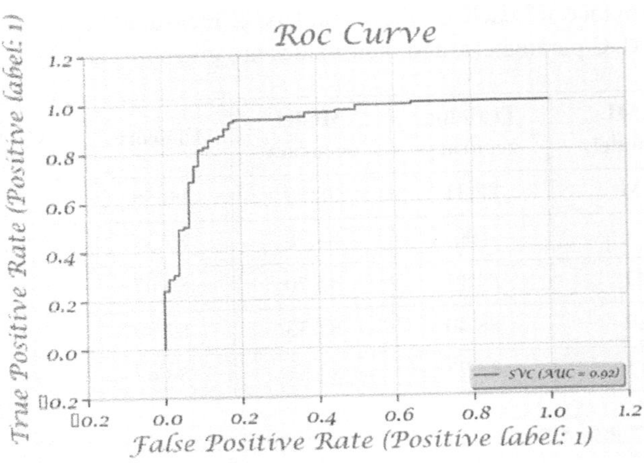

Figure 4.11. *ROC–AUC curve of the SVM model*

The performance comparison of ML models with the existing work is shown in Table 4.4. Parthiban and Srivatsa (2012) obtained an accuracy of 74% for HD detection using the NB model. Dwivedi et al. (2018) obtained an accuracy of 83% using the NB model and 82% using the SVM model for HD detection. Otoom et al. (2015) obtained an accuracy of 84.52% using the SVM model for HD detection. But our obtained ML models performed better as compared to other existing models for HD detection by using the fivefold cross-validation method.

Existing work	ML models	Accuracy
Proposed model	Naive Bayes	83.77%
	SVM	88.59%
	SGD	85.31%
	MLP	84.78%
	RF	86.41%

Table 4.4. *Performance comparison of the proposed model with the existing model*

4.8. Conclusion

The overarching goal of this research is to define several data mining algorithms that can effectively forecast cardiac disease. Our objective is to provide predictions that are accurate and efficient while using fewer features and tests. In this research, we only prioritized 12 essential characteristics. We used five data mining classification approaches, namely SVM, NB, MLP, SGD and RF. Among these five classification models, SVM gave the highest prediction accuracy of 88.52% and an AUC of 92.2%. This research can be expanded by including other used ML methods such as ensemble technique, clustering, bacteria foraging optimization technique, cat swarm optimization technique and association rules algorithm. Given the shortcomings of this study, there is a need to implement more sophisticated and combined models to improve the accuracy of the early prognosis of the heart condition.

4.9. References

Chang, V., Rupa Bhavani, V.R., Xu, A.Q., Hossain, M.A. (2022). An artificial intelligence model for heart disease detection using machine learning algorithms. *Healthcare Analytics*, 2, 100016.

Dev, S., Wang, H., Nwosu, C.S., Jain, N., Veeravalli, B., John, D. (2022). A predictive analytics approach for stroke prediction using machine learning and neural networks. *Healthcare Analytics*, 2, 100032.

Dwivedi, A.K. (2018). Performance evaluation of different machine learning techniques for prediction of heart disease. *Neural Computing & Applications*, 29(10), 685–693.

Guleria, P. and Sood, M. (2020). Intelligent learning analytics in the healthcare sector using machine learning. In *Machine Learning with Health Care Perspective*. Springer, Cham.

Martin-Isla, C., Campello, V.M., Izquierdo, C., Raisi-Estabragh, Z., Baeßler, B., Petersen, S.E., Lekadir, K. (2020). Image-based cardiac diagnosis with machine learning: A review. *Frontiers in Cardiovascular Medicine*, 7, 1. doi: 10.3389/fcvm.2020.00001.

Mehrang, S., Pietilä, J., Korhonen, I. (2018). An activity recognition framework deploying the random forest classifier and a single optical heart rate monitoring and triaxial accelerometer wrist-band. *Sensors*, 18(2), 613.

Mohapatra, R.K, Mishra, S., Azam, M., Dhama, K. (2021). COVID-19, WHO guidelines, pedagogy, and respite. *Open Medicine (Poland)*, 16(1), 491–493.

Mohapatra, R.K., Kuppili, S., Suvvari ,T.K., Kandi, V., Behera, A., Verma, S , Biswal, S.K., Al-Noor, T.H., El-ajaily MM, Sarangi, A.K. et al. (2022). SARS-CoV-2 and its variants of concern including Omicron: A never ending pandemic. *Chemical Biology & Drug Design*, 99(5), 769.

Muhammad, Y., Tahir, M., Hayat, M., Chong, K. (2020). Early and accurate detection and diagnosis of heart disease using intelligent computational model. *Scientifc Reports*, 10, 19747. doi: 10.1038/s41598-020-76635-9.

Nagavelli, U., Samanta, D., Chakraborty, P. (2022). Machine learning technology-based heart disease detection models. *Journal of Healthcare Engineering*, 7351061. doi: 10.1155/2022/7351061.

Noshad, Z., Javaid, N., Saba, T., Wadud, Z., Saleem, M.Q., Alzahrani, M.E., Sheta, O.E. (2019). Fault detection in wireless sensor networks through the random forest classifier. *Sensors*, 19(7), 1–21.

Otoom, A.F., Abdallah, E.E., Kilani, Y., Kefaye, A., Ashour, M. (2015). Effective diagnosis and monitoring of heart disease. *International Journal of Software Engineering & Applications*, 9(1), 143–156.

Pal, M., Parija, S., Mohapatra, R.K., Mishra, S., Rabaan, A.A, Al Mutair ,A., Alhumaid, S., Al-Tawfiq, J.A., Dhama, K. (2022a). Research article symptom-based COVID-19 prognosis through AI-based IoT: A bioinformatics approach. *BioMed Research International*. doi: 10.1155/2022/3113119.

Pal, M., Parija, S., Panda, G., Dhama, K., Mohapatra, R.K. (2022b). Risk prediction of cardiovascular disease using machine learning classifiers. *Open Med.*, 17(1), 1100–1113.

Parthiban, G. and Srivatsa, S.K. (2012). Applying machine learning methods in diagnosing heart disease for diabetic patients. *International Journal of Applied Information Systems (IJAIS)*, 3(7), 25–30.

Shah, D., Patel, S., Bharti, S.K. (2020). Heart disease prediction using machine learning techniques. *SN Computer Science*, 1, 345. doi: 10.1007/s42979-020-00365-y.

Wang, C. and Liang, C. (2018). Msipred: A python package for tumor microsatellite instability classification from tumor mutation annotation data using a support vector machine. *Scientific Reports*, 8(1), 1–10.

Zahariev, A., Zveryakov, M., Prodanov, S., Zaharieva, G., Angelov, P., Zarkova, S., Petrova, M. (2020). Debt management evaluation through support vector machines: On the example of Italy and Greece. *Entrepreneurship and Sustainability Issues*, 7(3), 1–12.

5

3D Volume Rendering of MRI Images for Tumor Detection and Segmentation using nnUnet

This chapter presents a comprehensive framework for segmentation and 3D model reconstruction of tumors (such as glioma) and the brain from MRI scans, using advanced techniques such as nnUnet and other algorithms. The methodology includes the segmentation of the MRI scan using nnUnet, merging the files and finally 3D reconstruction using vtk and itk libraries. The experimental evaluation demonstrates high accuracy and performance of nnUnet models, achieving excellent segmentation results. The 3D reconstruction with the marching cube algorithm produces realistic models that are exportable in popular formats. The proposed methodology offers a short processing time of approximately one minute and provides valuable 3D models for applications in 3D printing, augmented reality, mixed reality and medical research. The research highlights the potential of deep learning and advanced algorithms in medical image analysis and visualization.

5.1. Introduction

Millions of individuals are affected each year by brain tumors, which is one of the main causes of mortality and disability globally. For the purposes of diagnosis, planning treatments and keeping track of the course of the disease, brain tumors must be accurately segmented and diagnosed. The traditional method of brain tumor segmentation uses labor-intensive, subjective and often error-prone human or semi-automated procedures. This has spurred the creation of automated

Chapter written by Sai AYUSH, Sai Sreeram GADDE, RAJESWARI and Shivarudraiah SUMALATHA.
For a color version of all the figures in this chapter, see www.iste.co.uk/pradhan/cognitivecomputing.zip.

segmentation techniques that can deliver precise and effective segmentation outcomes.

Deep learning techniques have made significant progress in the segmentation of medical images in recent years. A deep learning architecture called Unet has attained state-of-the-art performance in a number of segmentation tasks. A variety of medical picture segmentation tasks, including those involving heterogeneous and irregularly shaped objects, can be trained on the highly adaptable architecture of Unet (Alqaoud et al. 2022).

This chapter discusses the work on segmenting the brain mask and a particularly diverse brain tumor called glioma, using Unet. The intrinsic heterogeneity of glioma, a particular type of brain tumor, makes segmenting it difficult due to three types of brain cells. Our strategy was inspired by the need for more precise and effective techniques for segmenting brain tumors, especially in the context of heterogeneous tumors, such as gliomas.

Unet is a popular deep learning architecture for medical image segmentation. nnUnet is a framework developed for using the Unet algorithm Since its debut in 2018, it has gained popularity as a method for segmenting medical images, generating cutting-edge results on a variety of segmentation tasks. A wide variety of medical picture segmentation tasks, including those involving heterogeneous and irregularly shaped objects, can be trained on with nnUnet, thanks to its extreme adaptability architecture and user-friendly framework.

The segmentation of medical images is made possible by the Unet architecture, which is built on a number of encoding and decoding blocks. While the decoding blocks create the segmentation mask by upsampling and concatenation operations, the encoding blocks use convolutional layers to extract features from the input image. Cross-entropy loss and Dice loss, which are frequently used in medical image segmentation, are combined to train the network.

The research includes the development and training of nnUnet models for the segmentation of gliomas and brain masks, as well as a demonstration of the viability of using the vtk and itk libraries to convert segmentation files into 3D models. The segmentation data are kept in the NIfTI format, which is often used in both clinical settings and medical imaging research. The vtk and itk libraries offer strong platforms for further analysis and investigation, and are effective tools for visualizing and analyzing 3D medical images.

A brief review of research on brain tumor segmentation and 3D reconstruction is presented in the following section. Furthermore, the process for developing the Unet models and creating the 3D models, the dataset that was used for training and testing, as well as the pre-processing procedures that were used to get the data ready for training are discussed. Finally, the experimental results and evaluation of the performance of the approach are shown.

This study demonstrates the potential of using 3D reconstruction and deep learning techniques in advancing the field of medical image segmentation. It highlights the effectiveness of nnUnet and 3D reconstruction algorithms in accurately and efficiently segmenting heterogeneous brain tumors and brain masks, resulting in the generation of a comprehensive 3D model. These findings offer valuable insights into medical image analysis, paving the way for further research and advancements in this area.

5.2. Methodology

The methodology is divided into three parts, using different algorithms, such as Unet, marching cube algorithm, etc. The input MRI scan is segmented using the first nnUnet model for brain masking and then a cropped MRI scan is generated; the cropped MRI scan is then used for detecting tumors and segmented using the second nnUnet model. These output segmentation files are overlapped together to form a single segmentation file using Python scripts. This segmentation file is further reconstructed into a 3D model using itk and vtk libraries.

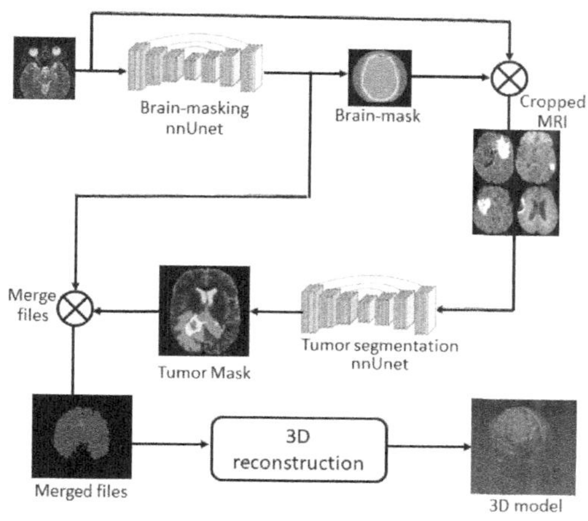

Figure 5.1. *Flow diagram*

5.2.1. *Segmentation*

The segmentation is performed using two trained Unet models that utilize the nnUnet framework. The two separate nnUnet models have unique architectures optimized for their specific task.

The first model was trained on the Calgary-Campinas-359 (CC-359) dataset. The Calgary-Campinas-359 (CC-359) dataset is a commonly used dataset in medical imaging research, particularly for brain imaging. It consists of 359 T1-weighted magnetic resonance imaging (MRI) scans of the brain, each with a resolution of 256x256x256 voxels. The dataset includes both normal brain images as well as images with tumors and other abnormalities, making it a valuable resource for researchers studying brain diseases and disorders. The primary purpose of this model was to perform brain masking and skull stripping, which involves removing all non-brain tissue from the MRI scan to isolate the brain region (Souza et al. 2018). For training the model, 200 scans were used that accurately segmented the brain from each slice of the MRI scan. We used a 2D Unet architecture to train this model, which is a popular and widely used architecture for image segmentation tasks. The model was trained for a total of 336 epochs. The output segmentation file is then used with the input MRI scan to generate a cropped MRI scan of the brain. This MRI scan shows the skull-stripped MRI scan, showing only the brain tissues.

The second model was trained on the BraTS 2020 dataset. The BraTS dataset includes MRI scans of different modalities, such as T1-weighted, T2-weighted and FLAIR images, as well as ground truth labels for the tumors. The ground truth labels are provided by expert radiologists who manually segment the tumor regions on the images. The dataset is organized into training, validation and testing sets, with each set containing images and corresponding ground truth labels. The dataset also includes preprocessed images that have been skull-stripped and bias-corrected, as well as raw images that can be used for more advanced preprocessing techniques. There are three masks present, as the tumor is intrinsically heterogeneous, i.e. glioma. The segmentations were mainly enhancing tumor, non-enhancing tumor and edema (Menze et al. 2015).

This model's primary task was to accurately segment the tumor from the surrounding brain tissue of the cropped MRI scan generated. To achieve this, a 3D full-resolution architecture was used, which has demonstrated superior performance on 3D medical imaging segmentation tasks. The model was trained for 200 epochs.

After training was completed, the trained models were applied to a previously unknown test dataset, which included MRI scans of patients with brain tumors. The output of the brain mask nnUnet model is a binary mask, while the output of the tumor segmentation nnUnet model has three masks.

5.2.2. *Overlapping the scans*

The tumor segmentation file and the brain mask segmentation file are merged into a single file by overlapping the tumor on the brain mask. Since the dimensions of both the files are the same as that of the input MRI scan, the overlapping procedure does not lead to errors.

This is implemented by a custom Python script using the NumPy and Nibabel libraries. The script takes the file paths of the brain mask segmentation and tumor segmentation files as input, and outputs a new brain mask segmentation file with the tumor overlaid.

First, the script loads the brain mask segmentation file and its data using the nib.load() and get_fdata() functions, respectively. It then loads the tumor segmentation file and its data in the same way. The overlapping voxels between the two segmentations are identified using the np.where() function.

Next, the script updates the brain mask segmentation data at the overlapping voxels by adding a discrete value to the corresponding voxels in the tumor segmentation data. This ensures that the tumor voxels are distinguishable from the brain mask voxels in the overlaid segmentation.

Finally, the script saves the updated brain mask segmentation data as a new NIfTI file using the nib.Nifti1Image() and nib.save() functions. The output file name can be specified by the user.

5.2.3. *3D reconstruction*

The final segmentation file is loaded using the ITK library and then converted to a VTK image. The VTK image is written to the disk in the MetaImage format using the vtkMetaImageWriter function.

Then, the marching cubes algorithm is applied to extract a surface mesh from the volume using the vtkMarchingCubes function. This algorithm creates an isosurface, i.e. a 3D surface representing a specific value of the input image. In this case, the isovalue is set to 1, which corresponds to the tumor region in the brain mask segmentation. The resulting surface mesh is stored in vtk_polydata.

Finally, the reconstructed surface mesh is written to the disk in the OBJ format using the vtkOBJWriter function.

5.3. Results and discussion

The nnUnet models trained have shown a loss function of −0.98 and −0.71 for the brain mask model and tumor segmentations model, respectively, while training. The time taken for each epoch is 3 mins and 5 mins for the brain mask model and tumor segmentation model. This is observed due to a large number of the diverse dataset used in the tumor segmentation model, compared to the brain mask model. It is also due to the different architecture used for each application.

The training loss, validation loss and average global foreground Dice (for each segment) are presented in Table 5.1, for both the trained nnUnet models.

nnUnet model	Loss functions		
	Train loss	***Validation loss***	***Average global foreground Dice***
Tumor segmentation model	−0.7186	−0.6576	0.8473, 0.6967, 0.8688
Brain mask model	−0.9804	−0.9762	0.988

Table 5.1. *Loss functions*

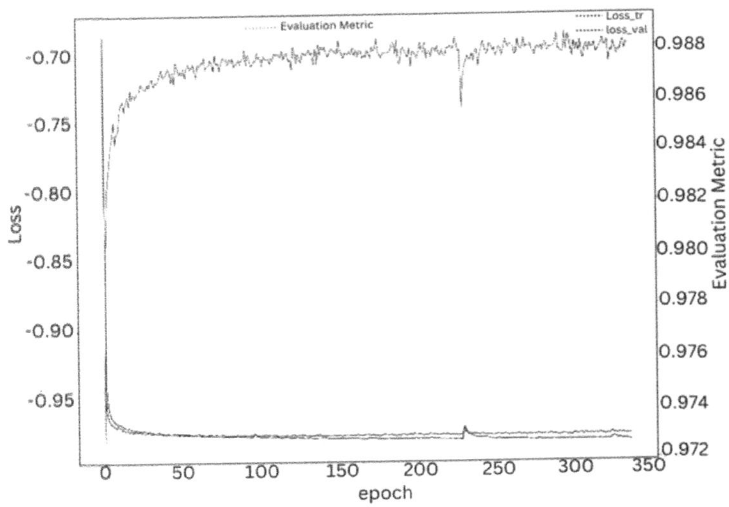

Figure 5.2. *Loss function – skull stripping*

The progress of loss functions appears to be decreasing substantially for every epoch and increasing the accuracy levels. The dataset trained contains a variety of patient data, depending on age, sex and health conditions, hence a diverse dataset leading to loss function decreasing.

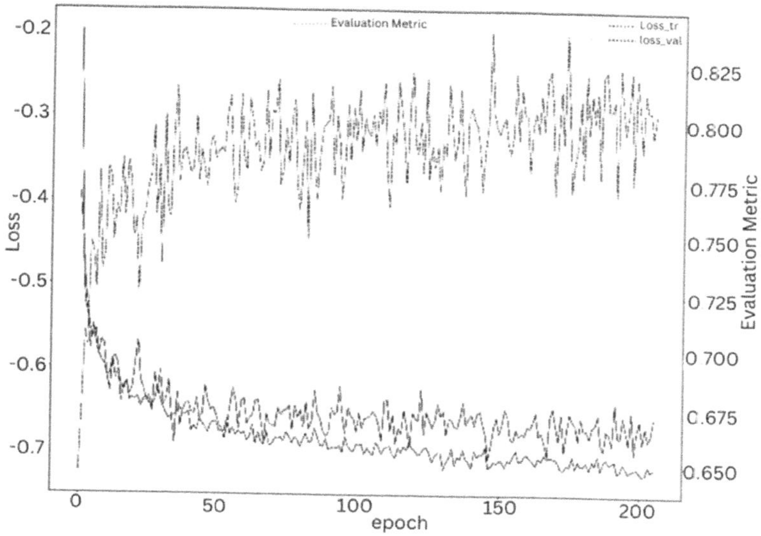

Figure 5.3. *Loss function – tumor segmentation*

The performance metrics of the segmentation models are observed and tabulated. The performance metrics are calculated by comparing the segmentation outputs with the ground truth segments manually provided by medical professionals.

nnUnet model	**Performance metrics**				
	Accuracy	**Dice**	**Jaccard**	**Precision**	**Recall**
Tumor segmentation model	0.998	0.999	0.998	0.998	0.999
Brain mask model	0.972	0.986	0.9728	0.977	0.994

Table 5.2. *Performance metrics*

These segmentations are in NIfTI files and have the same dimensions as the MRI scans. Hence, these can be used for the next step, which is overlapping into one file.

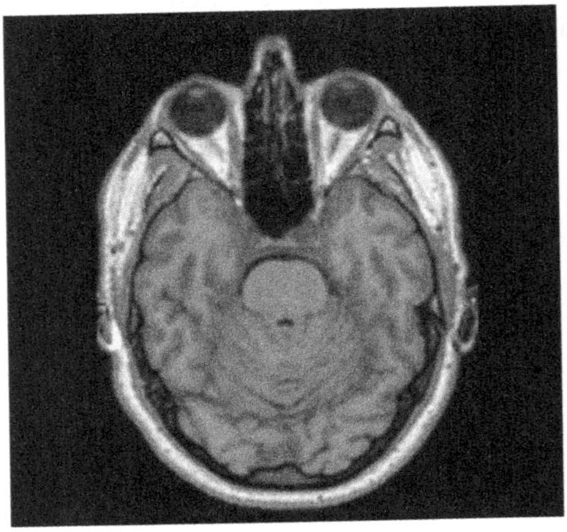

Figure 5.4. *MRI scan*

During the merging or overlapping of the tumor masks onto the brain mask, the probability of errors occurring is very low, which is due to the same dimensions of the scan as the input MRI scan. The accuracy level is dependent on the nnUnet output segmentation file generated.

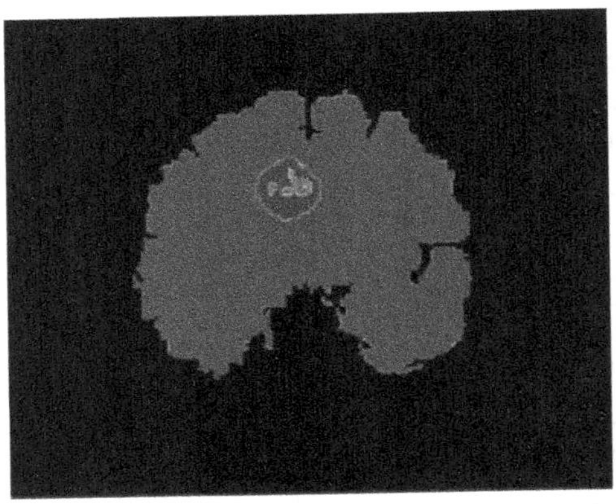

Figure 5.5. *Segmentations*

The 3D model is generated using a marching cube algorithm using the itk and vtk libraries. This generated 3D model can be modified into an obj or stl file, depending on the user's needs.

The time taken for the segmentation of test cases from each nnUnet model is about 20 seconds, and the time taken for merging of files and reconstruction is about 30 seconds. Hence, the total time taken for the process of generating a 3D model from MRI scan takes about 1 minute using the proposed pipelined methodology.

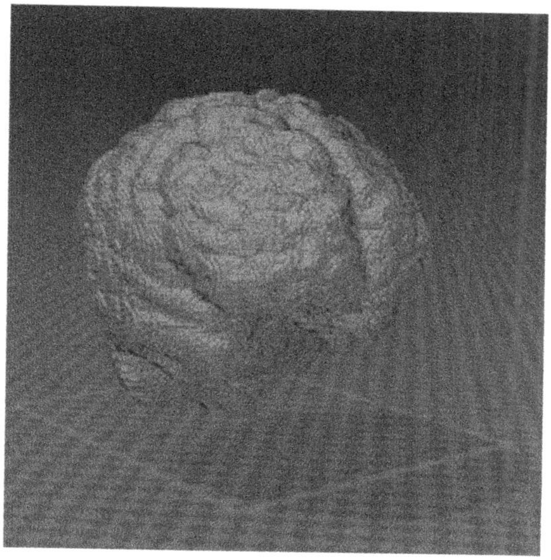

Figure 5.6. *3D model*

5.4. Conclusion and future scope

The proposed methodology is an effective method for adaptable custom segmentation and 3D reconstruction of the MRI scans using nnUnet and various other Python libraries. The process takes about one minute for generating a multi-model 3D object in an obj format, which can be used for several applications. The 2D segmentation file in NIfTI can also be accessed by the user for other medical or research purposes, which is supported in all medical applications. This chapter proposes an effectively formulated concept that can be applied to not only MRI but also CT scans. Future works include any modifications of nnUnet architectures such as SE-modified Unet architecture, which can be implemented for faster training time and faster prediction time. Providing a dataset that includes the brain mask and brain tumor in a file can eliminate the multiple steps proposed in this chapter. The itk and vtk libraries can be explored, and the 3D model reconstructed can be done with interpolations and smoothening factors for better resolution 3D models. The 3D models generated can be used for various further research and development such as using augmented reality and mixed reality for 3D model projection.

5.5. References

Aledhari, M. and Razzak, R. (2020). An adaptive segmentation technique to detect brain tumors using 2D Unet. *2020 IEEE International Conference on Bioinformatics and Biomedicine (BIBM)*, Seoul, 2328–2334. doi: 10.1109/BIBM49941.2020.9313547.

Alqaoud, M., Plemmons, J., Feliberti, E., Dong, S., Kaipa, K., Fichtinger, G., Xiao, Y., Audette, M.A. (2022). nnUNet-based multi-modality breast MRI segmentation and tissue-delineating phantom for robotic tumor surgery planning. *2022 44th Annual International Conference of the IEEE Engineering in Medicine & Biology Society (EMBC)*, Glasgow, 3495–3501. doi: 10.1109/EMBC48229.2022.9871109.

Bakas, S., Akbari, H., Sotiras, A., Bilello, M., Rozycki, M., Kirby, J.S., Freymann, J.B., Farahani, K., Davatzikos, C. (2017). Advancing the cancer genome atlas glioma MRI collections with expert segmentation labels and radiomic features. *Nature Scientific Data*, 4, 170117. doi: 10.1038/sdata.2017.117.

Bakas, S., Reyes, M., Jakab, A., Bauer, S., Rempfler, M., Crimi, A., Shinohara, R.T., Berger, C., Ha, S.M., Rozycki, M. et al. (2018). Identifying the best machine learning algorithms for brain tumor segmentation, progression assessment, and overall survival prediction in the BRATS challenge. arXiv preprint arXiv:1811.02629.

Dong, H., Xia, L., Zhang, J., Cai, A. (2013). Medical image reconstruction based on ITK and VTK. *2013 International Conference on Computer Sciences and Applications*, Wuhan, 642–645. doi: 10.1109/CSA.2013.155.

Isensee, F., Jaeger, P.F., Kohl, S.A., Petersen, J., Maier-Hein, K.H. (2021). nnU-Net: A self-configuring method for deep learning-based biomedical image segmentation. *Nature Methods*, 18(2), 203–211.

Menze, B.H., Jakab, A., Bauer, S., Kalpathy-Cramer, J., Farahani, K., Kirby, J., Burren, Y., Porz, N., Slotboom, J., Wiest, R. et al. (2015). The multimodal brain tumor image segmentation benchmark (BRATS). *IEEE Transactions on Medical Imaging*, 34(10), 1993–2024. doi: 10.1109/TMI.2014.2377694.

Souza, R., Lucena, O., Garrafa, J., Gobbi, D., Saluzzi, M., Appenzeller, S., Rittner, L., Frayne, R., Lotufo, R. (2018). An open, multi-vendor, multi-field-strength brain MR dataset and analysis of publicly available skull stripping methods agreement. *Neuroimage*, 170, 482–494. doi: 10.1016/j.neuroimage.2017.08.021.

Suri, J.S., Bhagawati, M., Agarwal, S., Paul, S., Pandey, A., Gupta, S.K., Saba, L., Paraskevas, K.I., Khanna, N.N., Laird, J.R. et al. (2022). UNet deep learning architecture for segmentation of vascular and non-vascular images: A microscopic lock at UNet components buffered with pruning, explainable artificial intelligence, and bias. *IEEE Access*, 11, 595–645. doi: 10.1109/ACCESS.2022.3232561.

6

Implementation of Key Generation in Kyber for Post-Quantum Cryptography using VIVADO

Quantum cryptography is a field that creates secure channels of communication between two parties by applying the ideas of quantum mechanics. It uses the principles of physics to secure information, in contrast to classical encryption, which is based on mathematical techniques. Due to the potential risk that quantum computers pose to conventional encryption techniques, post-quantum cryptography is an important area of research. A proposed post-quantum method for ensuring secure key exchange and encryption is the Kyber cryptographic system. It is built to survive both classical and quantum attacks and is based on the learning-with-errors (LWE) problem. Kyber provides a range of security levels and exhibits remarkable efficiency in key generation, encryption and decryption developments in the study of post-quantum cryptography.

The main goal of this work is to analyze the Kyber scheme thoroughly, with a focus on the simulation of the key generation block using register transfer level (RTL) design. In particular, for the Kyber768 variant, the simulation demonstrates the key generation block's functionality. This chapter shows the applicability of Kyber in practice and lays the groundwork for future developments in post-quantum cryptography research by implementing the algorithm and simulating its key generation block in RTL.

Chapter written by Srinivasa Murthy OMKAR, Siddabassappa Manjunath SUJAN, RAJESWARI and Shivarudraiah SUMALATHA.

For a color version of all the figures in this chapter, see www.iste.co.uk/pradhan/cognitivecomputing.zip.

6.1. Introduction

Traditional cryptography techniques rely on mathematical puzzles that are challenging to answer, including factoring big numbers or computing discrete logarithms. Many of the cryptographic techniques currently in use could be made vulnerable to attacks using Shor's algorithm and the development of quantum computing. Many of the present encryption techniques could become obsolete because quantum computers are able to solve these issues much faster than traditional computers. New encryption algorithms must be created to defend against attacks from quantum computers (Bisheh-Niasar et al. 2021).

PQC is a developing area of study that examines the possible danger that quantum computers pose to established cryptography techniques. The primary goal of PQC research is to create new cryptographic algorithms based on issues that are thought to be challenging, even for quantum computers. With a level of security that can withstand attacks from quantum computers, these algorithms represent a possible replacement for conventional encryption techniques.

Kyber is a post-quantum cryptography system that has drawn a lot of interest recently as a potential response to the security issues brought on by quantum computing. It uses a key encapsulation mechanism (KEM) based on the hardness of the learning-with-errors (LWE) problem, which is thought to make it immune to attacks from both classical and quantum computers. It has undergone considerable research and evaluation by the cryptographic community, and has been chosen as a finalist in the National Institute of Standards and Technology's (NIST) effort to standardize post-quantum cryptography (Nguyen et al. 2022).

In this chapter, the work on the KYBER key generation block is discussed, which creates the secret key and the public key needed for secure communication between two parties. Using RTL (Register Transfer Level) language, the design and implementation of the Kyber key generating block is presented in this work, along with an FPGA board implementation using VIVADO. The critical generation time, resource use and power consumption of the suggested design are assessed. The outcomes show that the suggested design is producing keys with the required key size for the Kyber algorithm. Here, variant Kyber768 is designed particularly for this chapter.

In the next section, a brief overview of the methodology of building a key generation block in Kyber is provided. The steps involved in building the block which generates the public and secret key of expected size are discussed. Furthermore, we present the experimental results, which include waveforms, synthesis and implementation report.

6.2. Methodology

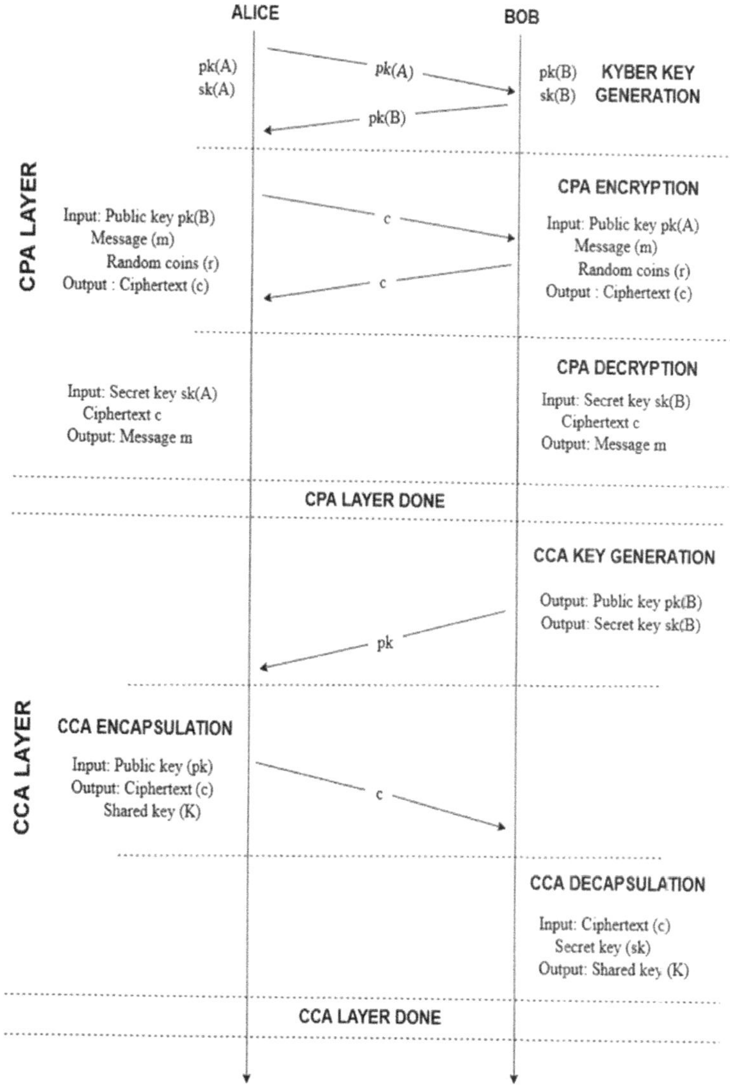

Figure 6.1. *Alice and Bob communication*

Kyber is a lattice-based PQC system that attempts to offer secure key exchange and public key encryption functionality. It is made for resistance to quantum computer attacks, which have the potential to compromise many established cryptography systems. This system, which incorporates components of both KEM and PKE, is adaptable and effective for creating secure communication in a post-quantum environment. It ensures data transmission's confidentiality and integrity, while providing security against both conventional and quantum adversaries.

The CPAPKE (Chosen-Plaintext Attack Public Key Encryption) technique developed by Kyber is made to be resistant against chosen-plaintext attacks, in which an attacker has access to encryption oracles and can ask for the encryption of particular plaintexts. The security of CPAPKE assures that even though an attacker has access to the public key and can watch the encryption of numerous plaintexts, they will not be able to obtain the private key or gather any relevant information.

In CCAKEM (Chosen-Ciphertext Attack Key Encapsulation Mechanism), the sender uses the recipient's public key to encapsulate a secret key, creating a ciphertext that can be sent securely. The shared secret key can then be extracted from the ciphertext by the recipient using the associated private key. The safety of CCAKEM assures that an attacker cannot discover any information about the shared secret key, even though they have access to encryption and decryption oracles and can perform chosen-ciphertext queries on them.

6.2.1. *RTL design*

The RTL simulation of the key generation block in Kyber involves designing and simulating the digital logic circuit that performs the key generation process. This block generates the secret and public keys used in the Kyber scheme. Here, RTL code for Kyber768 variant is designed specifically. The key generation block in Kyber768 involves several main blocks, such as a true random number generator (TRNG), Secure Hash Algorithm 3 (SHA3-512) function, pseudo-random number generator (PRNG), a number theoretic transform (NTT), and an encoding function. In this section, the methodology used to implement these blocks in RTL language is described.

6.2.2. *True random number generator and (SHA-512) HASH*

The first step in the key generation process is to obtain random numbers using the TRNG module. The TRNG module is used to generate a random number as the initial stage in the key creation process. The TRNG uses a physical phenomenon, such as noise being generated from an oscillator, as its entropy to produce a stream of random bits. The stream of valid random numbers is stored in FIFO, which then sends it into an FSM controlling the HASH module. The SHA3-512 module receives the valid random number that was generated by the TRNG, and it generates a hash digest that is of 512-bits in length. With the assistance of the slicer IP, this hash value is cut in half, producing the halves rho and sigma, respectively.

6.2.3. *Pseudo random number generator*

The PRNG module generates a series of pseudo-random numbers by using rho and sigma as seed input. In the Kyber key exchange protocol, these numbers are used to generate the matrix_A, the secret message and the error vector. Sigma is used to generate the secret vector and error vector matrices, which is of size kx1, and Rho is used to generate the matrix_A, which is of size k x k. In this instance, k=3. The 12-bit output required for matrix generation is provided by the FSM used in this case.

6.2.4. *Numeric theoretic transform*

The NTT module then processes the matrix_A and secret matrix by applying the Number Theoretic Transform to the vector of matrix to convert it from the time domain to the frequency domain. This NTT module was created especially for Kyber to achieve fast and efficient multiplication. The prime number chosen here is q = 3,329, which is used for all the calculations for performing modulo q operations. Also, the n = 256 is for all levels of Kyber, meaning the NTT module will take input of only 256 elements in the time domain and output the same 256 elements in the frequency domain.

The main purpose of using an NTT module to convert the matrices from the time domain to the frequency domain is to reduce the overall number of multiplications required, which will be required for further mathematical operations, such as matrix multiplication.

6.2.5. *Matrix multiplication*

After obtaining matrix A and s in the NTT domain, pointwise multiplication is performed for matrix multiplication in the frequency domain, which is required to multiply all 256 elements of matrix_A with other 256 elements of matrix_s.

Pointwise multiplication is accomplished by using the same NTT block. Here, the block performs both multiplication and INTT to multiply the data and return them to the time domain modulo q. Further resultant t is obtained by adding e to the resultant matrix. Finally, the polynomial representation, i.e. resultant t and s is passed through the encoding function to produce the encoded public and private keys, which are in byte format. Furthermore, in preparation for the key exchange procedure, the encoded keys are kept in memory or an FIFO.

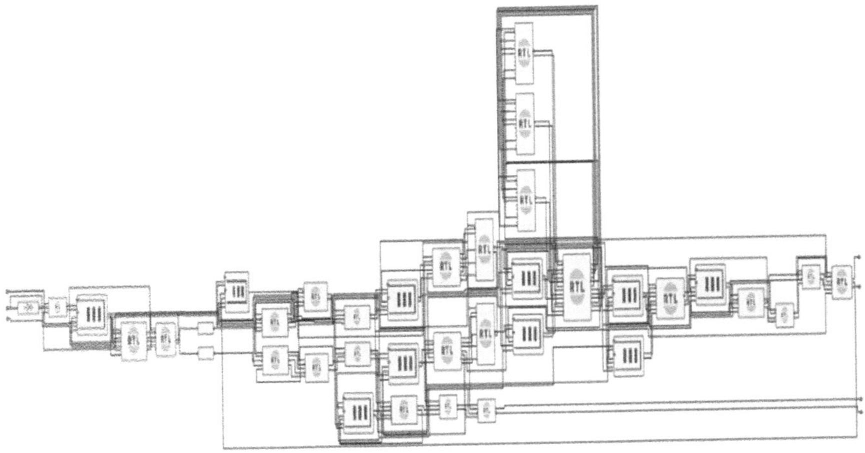

Figure 6.2. *RTL block design*

6.3. Results and discussion

6.3.1. *Design outcomes*

Public key and secret key with the requisite size are the results of the design process. The key is embodied in the valid signals. Figure 6.4 represents the pk generation of size 9,472 bits.

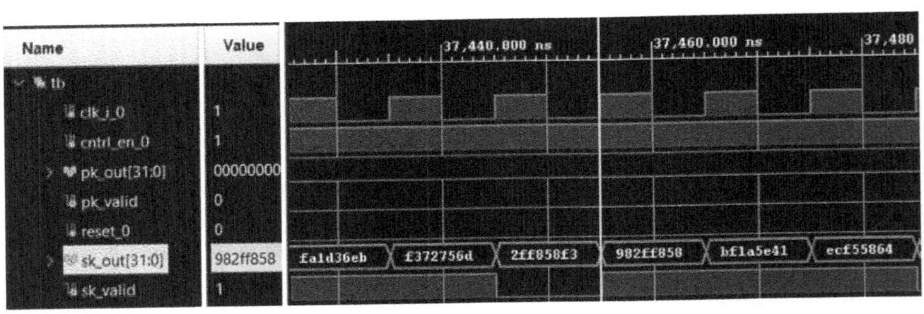

Figure 6.3. *sk generation*

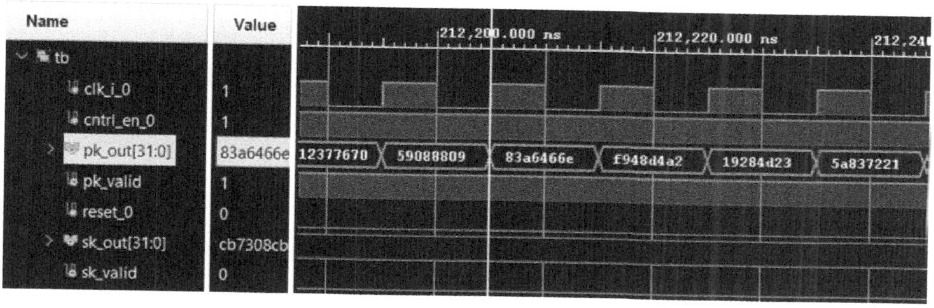

Figure 6.4. *pk generation*

6.3.2. *Board specifications*

The Kria KV260 Vision AI Starter Kit is a development platform for Kria K26 SOMs built for advanced vision application development, without requiring complex hardware design knowledge.

The dimensions of the Kria KV260 Vision AI Starter Kit are 119 mm x 140 mm x 36 mm and weight of 205 g. The KV260 features multi-camera support through 2x on semi-image access system (IAS) connectors and 1x Raspberry Pi connector. The kit also includes flexible I/O connectivity through Ethernet, USB and JTAG.

6.3.3. *Interfacing with processor core using AXI*

Once the key generation block is finished being designed, a hierarchy is created. The output port is first linked to an AXI FIFO and then to DMA in order to quickly transport data.

The processor ZYNQ board, which manages data globally, is connected to the entire design. The processor can be managed by sending interrupts using the SDK (Software Development Kit).

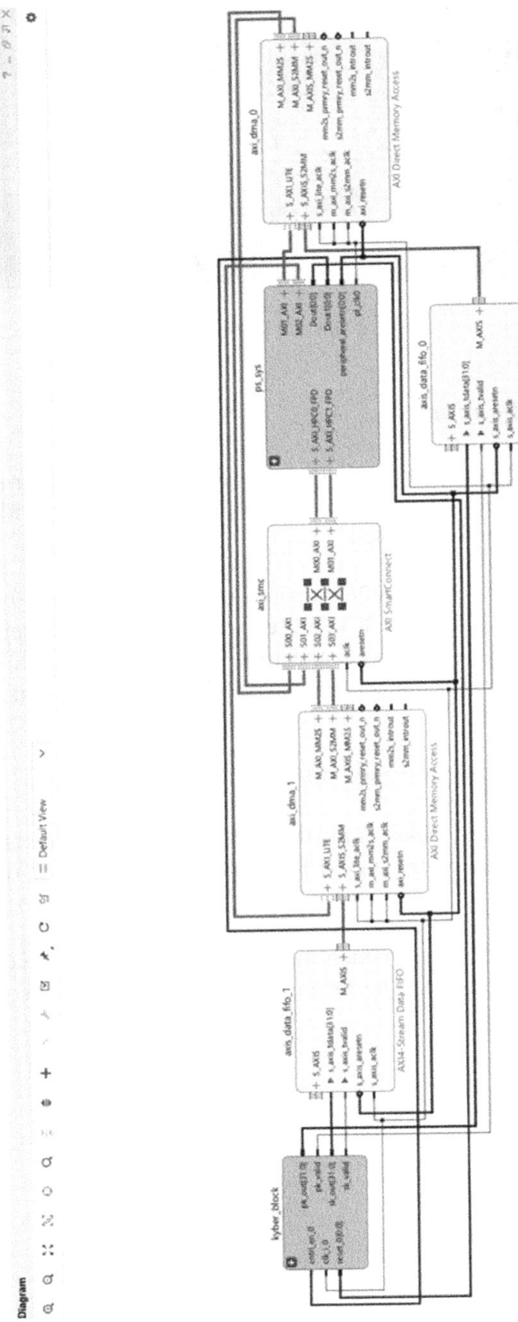

Figure 6.5. *A key generation implementation with processor subsystem*

RTL synthesis is a process in digital design where a high-level RTL description of a circuit is translated into a gate-level netlist that can be implemented in hardware.

The process involves mapping the RTL design onto specific hardware components such as lookup tables, registers and logic gates. The synthesized design is then optimized for timing, area and power.

RTL synthesis in Vivado produces a number of reports that provide information about the design's performance and resource usage. This report provides information about the design's timing constraints and the estimated timing performance of the design. It also includes detailed information about the resource usage in the design, including the number of LUTs, FFs, BRAMs and DSPs used. It also provides information about the usage of other resources, such as IOBs and BUFGs.

6.3.4. *Area utilization*

This section shows the number of LUTs (lookup tables) used in the FPGA's configurable logic blocks (CLBs). The table shows the following utilization outcomes:

a) LUT: 30.33% of the available LUTs have been used, with a total of 35,525 LUTs used. Of these, 33,711 LUTs are used as logic, while the remaining 1,814 LUTs are used as memory.

b) CLB registers: 22.41% of the available registers have been used, with a total of 52,502 registers used. Of these, 18,061 registers are used as flip-flops, while the remaining 34,441 registers are used as latches.

c) CARRY8: 1.56% of the available CARRY8 units have been used, with a total of 228 units used.

d) F7 Muxes, F8 Muxes and F9 Muxes: 7.61% of the available F7 Muxes have been used, with a total of 4,458 units used. Similarly, 7.24% of the available F8 Muxes have been used, with a total of 2,121 units used. No F9 Muxes have been used in this design.

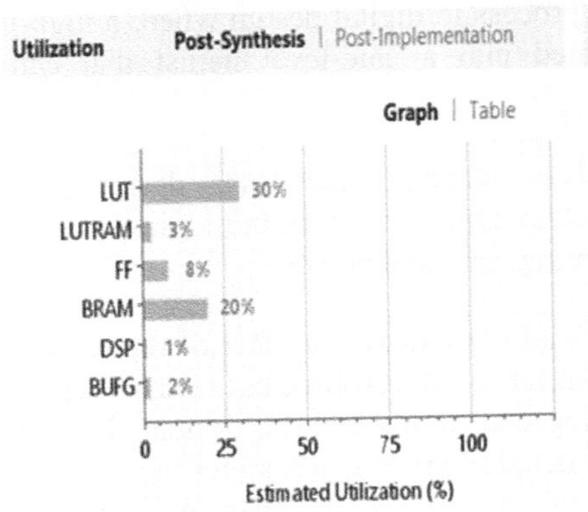

Figure 6.6. *Area utilization report (post-synthesis)*

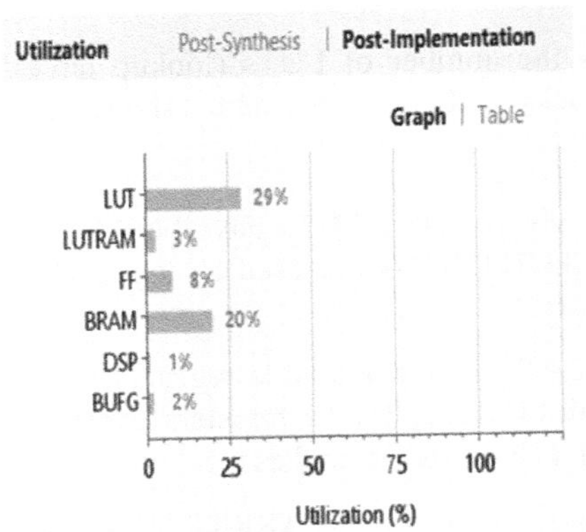

Figure 6.7. *Area utilization report (post-implementation)*

6.3.5. *Power utilization*

The Vivado power report gives critical information about a design's power usage on an FPGA. The total on-chip power for the design is 3.813 W. The junction temperature, which indicates the expected temperature at the core of the FPGA, is 33.8°C. The thermal margin, which represents the difference between the junction temperature and the maximum safe junction temperature, is 512°C, guaranteeing that the junction temperature remains considerably below the limit. The effective

OJA, which represents the thermal resistance of the FPGA package and its capacity to dissipate heat, is 2.3°C/W, demonstrating efficient heat dissipation capabilities.

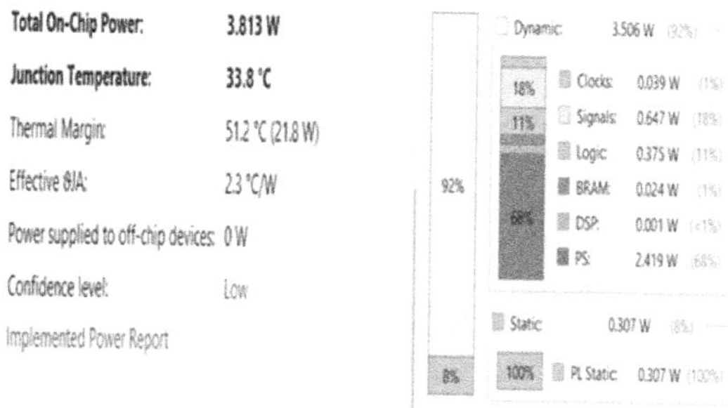

Figure 6.8. *Power utilization*

6.3.6. *Timing utilization*

The timing report generated by Vivado summarizes the timing analysis performed on the design. This consists of three sections: Setup, Hold and Pulse Width. In the Setup section, there are no timing violations, as indicated by a total negative slack (TNS) of 0 and zero failing endpoints. Similarly, the Hold section shows no hold violations, with a total hold slack (THS) of Ons and no failing endpoints. The Pulse Width section also reports no pulse width violations, with a total pulse width negative slack (TPWS) of Ons and no failing endpoints. Overall, the timing report confirms that the design meets its timing requirements, as there are no timing violations detected.

Timing	**Setup**
Worst Negative Slack (WNS):	2.805 ns
Total Negative Slack (TNS):	0 ns
Number of Failing Endpoints:	0
Total Number of Endpoints:	60650

Figure 6.9. *Setup report*

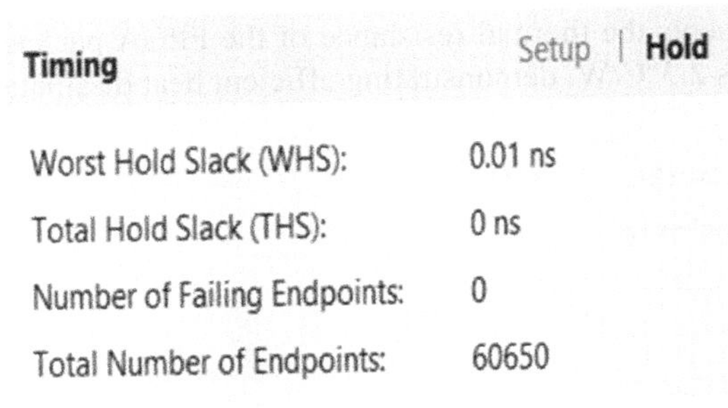

Figure 6.10. *Hold report*

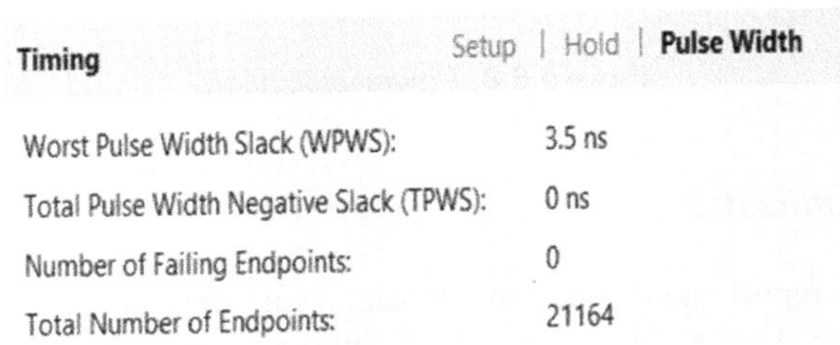

Figure 6.11. *Pulse width report*

6.4. Conclusion and future scope

The key generation block of Kyber PQC KEM in RTL. This version is tailored specifically for the Kyber768 variant, balancing performance and security characteristics to meet the needs. This work mainly involves building FSM between important components such as TRNG, PRNG, NTT block and Encoder to regulate data flow and pipelining between them in this design. It also meets the criteria of both public and secret keys by creating the required key size, respectively. The future scope includes developing an optimized Kyber module that meets the security-level specifications of Kyber PQC KEM. The Kyber key generation block tailored specifically for the Kyber768 variant is implemented, which generates the secret key and the public key needed for secure communication between two parties. Using RTL language, the design and implementation of the Kyber key generating block is presented in this work, along with an FPGA board implementation using Vivado. The critical generation time, resource use and power consumption of the suggested design are assessed. The outcomes show that the suggested design is producing keys with the required key size for the Kyber algorithm. Here, variant Kyber768 is designed particularly for this chapter.

6.5. References

Avanzi, R., Bos, J., Ducas, L., Kiltz, E., Lepoint, T., Lyubashevsky, V., Schanck, J.M., Schwabe, P., Seiler, G., Stehle, D. (2021). CRYSTALS-Kyber algorithm specifications and supporting documentation [Online]. Available at: https://pq-crystals.org/kyber/data/kyber-specification-round3-20210131.pdf.

Bertoni, G., Daemen, J., Peeters, M., Assche, G.V. (2013). Keccak and the SHA-3 standardization. NIST, Gaithersburg, MD [Online]. Available at: https://csrc.nist.gov/csrc/media/projects/hash-functions/documents/keccak-slides-at-nist.pdf.

Bisheh-Niasar, M., Azarderakhsh, R., Mozaffari-Kermani, M. (2021). Instruction-set accelerated implementation of CRYSTALS-Kyber. *IEEE Trans. Circuits Syst. I, Reg. Papers*, 68(11), 4648–4659.

Borges, F., Reis, P., Pereira, D. (2020). A comparison of security and its performance for key agreements in post-quantum cryptography. *IEEE Access*, 8, 142413–142422. doi: 10.1109/ACCESS.2020.3013250.

Nguyen, T.T., Kim, S., Eom, Y., Lee, H. (2022). Area-time efficient hardware architecture for CRYSTALS-Kyber. *Appl. Sci.*, 12, 5305. doi: 10.3390/app12115305.

Pablos, J.I.E., Marriaga, M.E., Pozo, Á.L.P.d. (2022). Design and implementation of a post-quantum group authenticated key exchange protocol with the LibOQS library: A comparative performance analysis from classic McEliece, Kyber, NTRU, and Saber. *IEEE Access*, 10, 120951–120983. [Online]. Available at: https://ieeexplore.ieee.org/stamp/stamp.jsp?arnumber=9950501.

Pope, G. (n.d.). CRYSTALS-Kyber python implementation [Online]. Available at: https://github.com/GiacomoPope/kyber-py.

Putranto, D.S., Wardhani. R.W., Larasati, H.T., Kim, H. (2023). Space and time-efficient quantum multiplier in post quantum cryptography era. *IEEE Access*, 11, 21848–21862 [Online]. Available at: https://ieeexplore.ieee.org/stamp/stamp.jsp?arnumber=10058193.

Richter, M., Bertram, M., Seidensticker, J., Tschache, A. (2022). A mathematical perspective on post-quantum cryptography. *Mathematics*, 10, 2579. doi: 10.3390/math10152579.

Sim, B.-Y., Kwon, J., Lee, J., Kim, I.-J., Lee, T.-H., Han, J., Yoon, H., Cho, J., Han, D.-G. (2020). Single-trace attacks on message encoding in lattice-based KEMs. *IEEE Access*, 8, 183175–183191 [Online]. Available at: https://eprint.iacr.org/2020/992.pdf

7

Computational Intelligence and Big Data Analytics for Smart Healthcare: A Comprehensive Study

Computational intelligence techniques such as artificial intelligence, machine learning and data analytics are being increasingly applied in healthcare for improved diagnosis, treatment, patient engagement and administrative tasks. These technologies allow analysis of large, complex datasets from electronic health records, medical images, genomic data, wearables, etc. to uncover hidden insights and patterns. This enables personalized medicine, early disease detection, predictive analytics, optimized workflows and better resource allocation. This shows that AI can perform as well or better than humans at certain healthcare tasks such as diagnosing diseases using medical images. However, successful real-world implementation faces challenges such as integrating AI into clinical workflows, lack of large labeled training datasets, regulatory approval and ethical concerns around accountability and transparency. The concept of "smart healthcare" emerged in recent years as a result of the convergence of artificial intelligence and Big Data analytics in the healthcare industry. This chapter examines how these two fields interact and how they can be used to enhance healthcare results. It explores the methodology, techniques and difficulties associated with using Big Data analytics and computational intelligence for a variety of functions in smart healthcare, such as patient diagnostics, treatment optimization, disease prediction and improvement of operational efficiency.

Chapter written by Bhawna KAUSHIK and Mayank SAINI.

For a color version of all the figures in this chapter, see www.iste.co.uk/pradhan/cognitive computing.zip.

7.1. Introduction

Healthcare generates vast amounts of heterogeneous data from sources such as hospitals, insurance, medical research, wearables and more. There is huge potential to harness this Big Data using computational intelligence approaches like AI, machine learning and advanced analytics. These technologies allow the processing of complex data to derive actionable insights for improving healthcare delivery across prevention, diagnosis, treatment, patient engagement and administration. The fusion of computational intelligence, which encompasses artificial intelligence (AI), machine learning (ML) and optimization techniques, with Big Data analytics has paved the way for transformative advancements in healthcare. Smart healthcare leverages these technologies to enable data-driven decision-making, personalized treatment plans and predictive models for early disease detection.

7.1.1. *Computational intelligence in smart healthcare*

– Artificial intelligence in diagnostics: utilization of AI for image analysis and interpretation in radiology and pathology. Natural language processing (NLP) for extracting insights from electronic health records and medical literature. AI-driven expert systems for differential diagnosis and treatment recommendation.

– Machine learning for predictive analytics: predicting disease outbreaks and patient readmissions. Early diagnosis of chronic diseases through feature-rich patient profiles. Risk assessment and personalized intervention strategies.

– Optimization techniques for treatment planning: genetic algorithms for optimizing treatment parameters. Patient-specific treatment planning through mathematical optimization. Resource allocation and scheduling in healthcare facilities.

7.1.2. *Big Data analytics in smart healthcare*

– Electronic health records (EHRs) and health information exchange (HIE): integration of heterogeneous data sources for comprehensive patient profiles.

– Wearable devices and remote monitoring: analysis of continuous patient-generated data from wearables. Real-time monitoring for chronic disease management.

– Social media and patient sentiment analysis: extracting patient experiences and sentiments from social media platforms. Enhancing patient engagement and satisfaction.

7.1.3. *Challenges and future directions*

– Data security and privacy: ensuring the confidentiality of sensitive patient data. Implementing robust encryption and access control mechanisms.

– Ethical considerations: balancing the benefits of data analytics with patient privacy concerns. Addressing biases in AI models to ensure equitable healthcare.

– Integration of emerging technologies: incorporating blockchain for secure data sharing and provenance. Exploring the potential of edge computing for real-time analytics.

– Regulatory and legal frameworks: navigating healthcare regulations such as HIPAA and GDPR. Establishing guidelines for responsibility.

7.1.4. *The landscape of smart healthcare*

The meaning of "smart healthcare" and its definition, IoT, Big Data analytics, AI and other essential technologies are briefly described here. It has the significance of data science in generating insights for healthcare improvement. A strong synergy overview of computational intelligence and its use in healthcare are discussed. AI provides solutions for decision support and diagnosis. It has the applications of machine learning in patient risk assessment and disease prediction. There are techniques for resource allocation and treatment planning optimization. It uses finding insights using electronic health records (EHRs) to gain insights from data. There is the importance of interoperability when interchanging healthcare data. Remote patient monitoring and wearable technology involves creating ongoing patient data and taking information on patient experiences and feelings from social media. It provides a description of the Internet of Things (IoT) and its function in the healthcare industry. It uses remote patient monitoring and connected medical equipment, collecting real-time data to create individualized treatment strategies. It has smart settings and residences that support healthcare requirements. It has the idea of smart cities and how they can affect healthcare. It provides healthcare services integration within a smart city framework and urban planning based on data for effective healthcare delivery. It provides case studies of smart city healthcare programs that were effective. It juggles the use of data with patient security and privacy, and there are fairness and prejudice in AI model development. In a data-driven age, it has adherence to healthcare standards (HIPAA, GDPR). It provides useful implementations of illness early detection using Big Data analytics and AI. For cancer patients, it has individualized treatment plans. Chronic illnesses are remotely monitored to enhance patient outcomes. There are emerging technologies and partnerships. It has the function of blockchain in safe data exchange of health, real-time healthcare analytics with edge computing and collaboration between technology and healthcare professionals. It develops healthcare's future recap of how technology has revolutionized the healthcare industry, highlights the significance of ethical and responsible technology integration and imagines a time when everyone can access and benefit from smart healthcare.

7.2. Computational intelligence techniques in healthcare

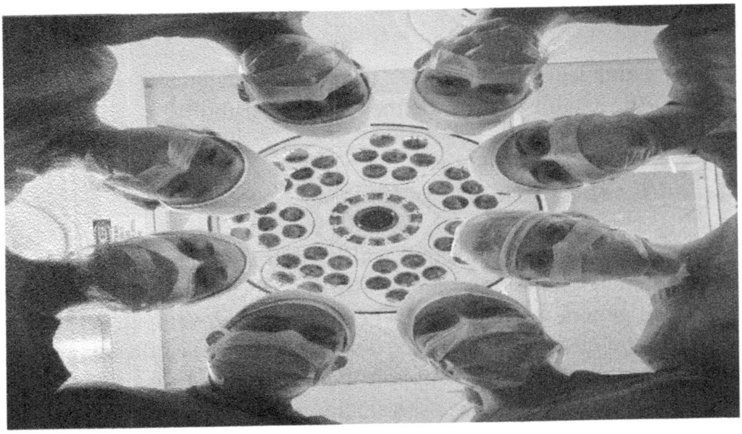

Figure 7.1. *Computational intelligence techniques in healthcare*

7.2.1. *Machine learning*

It identifies patterns in data to make predictions. It is used for precision medicine, image analysis and population health risk models. Machine learning has made significant contributions to the healthcare industry by leveraging computational techniques to analyze and extract valuable insights from medical data. Here are some key areas where machine learning is being applied in healthcare:

– Medical image analysis: machine learning algorithms, particularly deep learning models, have shown remarkable performance in interpreting medical images such as X-rays, MRIs and CT scans. They can assist in detecting anomalies, tumors, fractures and other abnormalities in medical images, aiding radiologists and clinicians in diagnosis.

– Disease diagnosis and prediction: machine learning models can analyze patient data, including medical records, lab results and genetic information, to assist in diagnosing diseases. They can also predict the likelihood of diseases based on patient characteristics, contributing to early intervention and personalized treatment.

– Drug discovery and development: by anticipating molecular interactions, finding prospective drug candidates and optimizing pharmacological characteristics, machine learning speeds up the drug discovery process. This shortens the time and expense needed to introduce new medications to the market.

– Personalized treatment plans: algorithms for machine learning can examine patient data to produce individualized treatment plans. Taking into account a person's genetic makeup and medical background, this involves figuring out the best drug dosages, how long to provide a course of treatment and any potential side effects.

– Genomic medicine: machine learning helps analyze genomic data to find genetic alterations linked to diseases, enabling early detection and individualized treatment plans.

– Health monitoring and wearables: wearable gadgets with sensors can continuously gather health information such as heart rate, level of exercise and sleep habits.

– Predictive analytics: by examining past data, machine learning algorithms can forecast patient outcomes, readmission risks and disease progression. This helps healthcare professionals make wise choices and allocate resources efficiently.

– Using natural language processing (NLP) techniques: computers are now able to comprehend and decipher human language. To facilitate effective data analysis and decision-making in the healthcare industry, NLP is used to extract information from clinical notes, medical reports and research papers.

– Healthcare management and fraud detection: machine learning is used to identify fraudulent activity in insurance and medical billing, lowering financial losses and enhancing overall healthcare management.

– Clinical studies and research: machine learning can help locate possible trial participants, match patients with appropriate studies and forecast patient reactions to certain medicines.

– Healthcare operations optimization: by anticipating patient admissions, resource allocation and staffing requirements, machine learning can enhance hospital operations and improve efficiency and patient care.

Machine learning can help with remote patient monitoring by evaluating data from wearable devices and notifying healthcare practitioners of any major changes in a patient's health. This is made possible by the development of telemedicine. The need for high-quality and diverse data, eliminating bias in models, protecting patient privacy and data security and negotiating legal and ethical considerations are just a few of the obstacles that still need to be overcome despite these achievements. Data scientists, healthcare practitioners, regulatory agencies and technological specialists must work together to achieve a safe and successful implementation of machine learning in healthcare.

7.2.2. *Natural language processing (NLP)*

It understands and classifies clinical notes, reports and other text data. It enables conversational AI. A subfield of artificial intelligence called "natural language processing" (NLP) is concerned with how computers and human language interact. In the field of healthcare, NLP is essential for deriving insightful information from unstructured clinical text data, including patient interviews, research papers, clinical notes and medical records. Here are some examples of how NLP is applied in the medical field:

– Clinical documentation and note processing: using natural language processing (NLP), structured information can be automatically extracted from free-text clinical notes, making it simpler for healthcare workers to examine and record patient data. This entails gathering information on diagnosis, therapies, drugs, allergies and other pertinent facts.

– Medical coding and billing: using clinical notes as a starting point, NLP can help generate correct medical codes and billing data, lowering errors and administrative demands on healthcare professionals.

– Clinical decision support: using NLP, systems can examine the clinical text and deliver pertinent data to help healthcare professionals make defensible decisions. For instance, NLP algorithms can highlight important patient data, alert possible drug interactions and provide recommendations for treatments based on scientific evidence.

– Drug and therapy information: NLP can extract data from databases and medical literature to give healthcare professionals the most recent details on medications, recommended courses of therapy and possible adverse effects.

– Research and literature analysis: NLP algorithms can examine a large volume of medical literature, research articles and clinical trials to pinpoint pertinent data, compile findings, and assist researchers in staying up to date with the most recent developments in their area of study.

– Sentiment analysis: to assess patient sentiment, contentment and worries, NLP can be used to evaluate patient evaluations, comments and social media posts. The patient experience can be enhanced by using this information by healthcare organizations.

– Disease surveillance and outbreak detection: NLP can keep an eye on news reports, social media posts and other sources to spot early indications of disease epidemics, assisting public health professionals in taking prompt action.

– Clinical trials matching: by examining patient profiles and trial requirements from clinical trial descriptions, NLP can assist in matching patients with the relevant clinical trials.

– Voice assistants and chatbots: NLP-driven virtual assistants and chatbots can give patients prompt answers to their questions about healthcare, as well as assist with making appointments, reordering prescriptions and giving out basic medical information.

– Translation services: NLP can help translate medical records and patient information into other languages, facilitating communication between patients who speak different languages and healthcare professionals.

– Risk prediction and early detection: NLP can examine patient records and notes to forecast the likelihood of developing particular illnesses, enabling healthcare professionals to take preventive steps and launch early therapies.

– Clinical research and data mining: for research purposes, NLP can be used to extract certain data from databases such as electronic health records, clinical trial data and other databases.

Medical jargon handling, adjusting to different linguistic styles and protecting patient data privacy and security are just a few of the difficulties NLP in healthcare encounters. To guarantee fair and accurate results, bias in data and algorithms is a serious issue that needs to be addressed. Despite these difficulties, NLP has great potential to improve the healthcare industry by enhancing patient care, accuracy and efficiency.

7.2.3. *Expert systems*

Rule-based clinical decision support is widely used in EHRs. However, there are limitations to maintaining complex rule sets. Expert systems in healthcare are computer-based systems that replicate the capability of human experts in a certain topic to make decisions. To offer suggestions, diagnoses and treatments in medical contexts, these systems make use of a combination of expertise in the domain, inference guidelines and logical reasoning. Expert systems are created to help medical practitioners by providing knowledge, recommendations and direction based on their expertise.

How expert systems are used in healthcare is as follows:

– Diagnosis and treatment: by reviewing test findings, medical history and patient symptoms, expert systems can help diagnose medical disorders. Based on accepted medical standards and best practices, they offer suggestions for additional examinations, therapies and interventions.

– Clinical decision support: during the course of treatment, healthcare providers can use expert systems as decision support tools. To help users make educated decisions, these systems provide information on drug interactions, possible adverse effects and available treatments.

– Educational resources: expert systems are used as educational resources by healthcare professionals, residents and medical students. To assist students in practicing diagnosis and treatment planning, they can offer case studies, simulations and scenarios.

– Medical procedures: medical procedures and guidelines can be continuously followed with the help of expert systems. They aid healthcare professionals in following established protocols, lowering the possibility of mistakes and enhancing patient outcomes. Expert systems can give healthcare professionals a second opinion, adding another level of validation to difficult diagnoses and treatment plans.

– Chronic disease management: by offering individualized care plans, medication reminders and lifestyle advice based on patient data, these systems can help in the management of chronic diseases.

Expert systems can assist remote healthcare providers in telemedicine situations by providing diagnostic assistance and treatment recommendations based on electronically supplied patient data. Expert systems can be used by researchers to analyze medical data, spot trends and produce ideas that can be tested further.

The following are the advantages of using expert systems in healthcare:

– Consistency: expert systems offer reliable, standardized advice that lowers the diversity in medical judgment.

– Access to knowledge: even in situations when specialist experts may not be readily available, healthcare professionals have access to a wide range of medical expertise and information.

– Efficiency: by processing and interpreting complicated medical data fast, expert systems reduce processing time.

– Reduced errors: expert systems can reduce medical errors by aiding in precise diagnosis and treatment planning.

– Continuous learning: by updating expert systems with the most recent medical guidelines and expertise, suggestions are always current.

Assuring that the expert system's knowledge base is correct and current, addressing any biases in decision-making, integrating these systems seamlessly into current healthcare processes and safeguarding patient privacy and data security are just a few of the challenges and factors to take into account. As technology develops, expert systems' capabilities can be improved by combining them with other AI methods like machine learning and natural language processing. This could lead to more efficient healthcare delivery.

7.2.4. *Robotic process automation (RPA)*

The term "robotic process automation" (RPA) refers to the use of software "bots" to automate repetitive and routine processes inside a business process. RPA is increasingly being used in healthcare to automate administrative processes, reduce manual work, reduce human errors and increase operational effectiveness. Here is an example of how RPA is used in the healthcare sector:

– Claims processing: by extracting data from claim forms, verifying the information, looking for errors and submitting claims to insurers, RPA can automate the processing of insurance claims. This shortens the claims procedure and lowers the possibility of mistakes.

– Billing and invoicing: RPA can automatically create invoices, charge patients and reconcile payments. This facilitates better revenue cycle management for healthcare providers.

– Scheduling appointments: RPA can handle scheduling, reminders and cancellations. To schedule appointments and identify open time slots, patients can communicate with bots.

– Data entry and integration: RPA can accurately and consistently enter patient data into electronic health records (EHR) systems. In addition, it can make it easier for databases and systems to integrate data.

– Automate the patient: RPA can automate the patient registration process, gathering relevant data and confirming insurance information.

– Medical coding and documentation: RPA can help with medical coding and documentation by assigning the proper medical codes to diagnoses and procedures to ensure accurate billing and payment. The documentation of patient visits can also be automated.

– Inventory supply: medical equipment, medication and supply inventory can all be managed using RPA, ensuring that stock levels are kept constant and orders are dispatched as needed.

– HR and payroll: RPA can automate a variety of human resources operations, including payroll processing, time and attendance monitoring and employee onboarding.

– Compliance and reporting: RPA can produce compliance reports to make sure healthcare firms follow legal and regulatory guidelines.

– Collection of data: healthcare companies can use RPA to collect data from a variety of sources for reporting and analysis, assisting them in making data-driven choices.

Patient outreach and follow-up: RPA can send pre-programmed reminders for prescription refills, follow-up visits and screenings.

Various advantages of RPA in healthcare are as follows:

– Efficiency: by removing manual and repetitive chores, RPA frees up healthcare staff to concentrate on more worthwhile endeavors.

– Accuracy: due to their high level of precision, bots are less likely to make mistakes when entering data, billing or coding.

– Cost savings: RPA increases overall operational efficiency while lowering labor expenses related to manual procedures.

– Consistency: RPA makes ensuring that jobs are carried out consistently by established guidelines and standards.

– Scalability: RPA can manage a large number of tasks without the need for more staff.

However, there are a few things to consider when using RPA in healthcare:

– Process standardization: RPA functions most effectively when procedures are clearly defined and uniform. It is possible that complex, unpredictable jobs are not fit for automation.

– Data security: RPA deals with private patient and financial information; therefore, maintaining data security and abiding by laws is crucial.

– Change management: to use RPA, workflows must be modified and personnel must be trained to collaborate with bots.

– Maintenance: to make sure they continue to operate properly, bots require regular maintenance, updates and monitoring.

RPA can greatly improve healthcare operations overall by lowering administrative burdens, enhancing accuracy and enabling healthcare workers to devote more time to patient care.

7.2.5. *Physical robots*

Physical robots are real, electromechanical machines that can be controlled by humans or operate autonomously. They are used in a variety of healthcare settings to help with patient care, clinical processes and operational effectiveness.

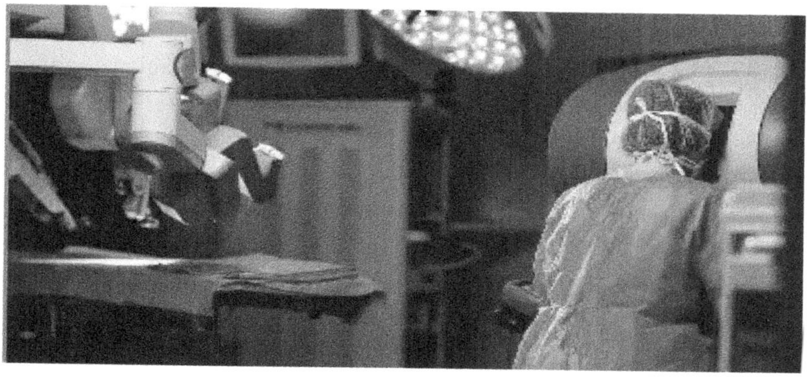

Figure 7.2. *Physical robots*

The following are some applications for physical robots in the healthcare sector:

– Surgical robots: surgeons can perform minimally invasive treatments with more accuracy and control thanks to surgical robots. These robots provide a 3D view of the surgical site and improve the surgeon's dexterity while lowering tremors. A good example is the da Vinci Surgical System, which is used for operations including hysterectomies and prostatectomies.

– Rehabilitation robots: patients with movement disabilities brought on by accidents, strokes or other illnesses benefit from the recuperation and physical therapy provided by rehabilitation robots. To increase strength, coordination and range of motion, these robots lead patients through exercises and offer feedback.

– Telepresence robots: telepresence robots allow medical practitioners work from a distance and communicate with patients and other healthcare workers. With the aid of their cameras, screens and audio systems, these robots can conduct remote real-time inspections and communications while also bridging geographic distances.

– Delivery robots: robots that transport meals, supplies and prescriptions to patients and healthcare workers are used in several hospitals and healthcare facilities. These robots use sensors to detect impediments as they go through hallways.

– Social robots: in environments such as long-term care institutions or elder care facilities, social robots provide emotional support and companionship to patients. These robots can converse, play games and give medicine and appointment reminders.

– Laboratory robots: robots used in laboratories automate tasks including handling, pipetting and sample preparation. In clinical laboratories, these robots increase precision, uniformity and throughput.

– Pharmacy robots: pharmacy robots automate the packaging, sorting and dispensing of medications. They make sure that medications are administered correctly, cut down on mistakes and give pharmacists more time.

– Disinfection robots: robotic disinfection systems – these systems use UV-C light or other technologies to sterilize surroundings and surfaces, assisting in reducing the transmission of diseases and infections in healthcare settings.

– Assistive robots: assistive robots assist with daily activities such as dressing, eating and bathing for those with disabilities or restricted mobility.

– Fall detection and prevention: robots with sensors can monitor patients and spot falls or strange movements, notifying caretakers or medical staff and allowing them to provide immediate assistance.

The following are the advantages of using physical robots in healthcare:

– Precision: robots can complete jobs with high accuracy, reducing the chance of human error.

– Remote accessibility: telepresence robots make medical consultations and care delivery possible at a distance, enhancing access to healthcare services.

– Safety: robots can handle potentially dangerous or infectious materials, lowering the dangers to healthcare staff.

– Repetitive tasks: robots are excellent at completing repetitive tasks reliably and without becoming weary.

– Enhanced patient experience: social robots and companion robots help patients feel less alone by offering emotional support.

The cost of acquisition and maintenance, potential staff and patient opposition, assuring adequate operation and maintenance training and addressing ethical and privacy concerns around patient engagement and data security are some of the challenges. As technology develops, the incorporation of physical robots with other technologies such as artificial intelligence (AI), machine learning and sensor networks will probably further increase the use of robots in improving patient outcomes and healthcare delivery.

7.3. Applications of intelligence and Big Data analytics in healthcare

Clinical decision support:

– AI algorithms can analyze patient medical records, lab tests and medical imaging data to suggest possible diagnoses and treatment options and predict outcomes.

– This assists physicians in making data-driven clinical decisions and identifying optimal treatments for patients.

– Several AI-based clinical decision support systems such as IBM Watson Health, Ada Health and Zebra Medical Vision have been developed.

Early disease detection and predictive analytics:

– Data mining techniques help identify patients at high risk of developing certain diseases such as diabetes and cardiovascular disease before symptoms appear.

– This enables preventive interventions. Machine learning models can also predict the likelihood of hospital readmission, sepsis onset, etc.

Precision medicine:

– Analyzing patient genetics, lifestyle, environment and biometrics data enables customizing diagnosis and treatments to the individual.

– For example, AI is used to analyze tumor genomic profiles to identify targeted therapies based on specific cancer molecular characteristics.

Patient monitoring and wearables:

– Wearable devices and sensors that continuously collect patient data such as heart rate and blood pressure enable real-time monitoring of vital parameters.

– AI techniques help analyze this data to flag risks and deterioration in health.

Population health management:

– Big Data analytics helps identify disease patterns and health trends across populations.

– This is used to guide public health policies, design preventive health programs and lower overall healthcare costs.

Operational and administrative analytics:

– AI and data science techniques are used to optimize clinical and administrative workflows, supply chains and resource allocation.

– This helps reduce healthcare costs and medical errors. Chatbots and virtual assistants are used for automating tasks.

7.4. Benefits of computational intelligence and Big Data analytics in healthcare

– Improved clinical outcomes and quality of care due to data-driven decisions and personalized treatments.

– Lower healthcare costs through optimized workflows, precision care and early interventions.

– Accelerated biomedical and healthcare research because of faster analysis of large datasets.

– Increased patient engagement and satisfaction through monitoring devices, chatbots and personalized care.

– Reduced medical errors and adverse events through continuous analytics-based patient monitoring.

– Enhanced accessibility and affordability of quality healthcare due to productivity improvements.

7.5. Challenges in implementing computational intelligence and Big Data analytics

– Poor data quality, inconsistencies, errors and missing data can compromise analytics and AI model accuracy.

– Interoperability issues and lack of data standards impede effective aggregation of health data across systems.

– Privacy and security concerns due to the use of personal patient data. It must comply with regulations like HIPAA.

– Physician acceptance and changing workflows are difficult. There is a lack of skills in interpreting the outputs of AI systems.

– Regulatory requirements for approving AI-based software as medical devices create barriers.

– Potential for bias and lack of transparency in data and algorithms leading to unfair outcomes.

7.6. Future aspect of computational intelligence and Big Data analytics in smart healthcare

Computational intelligence (CI) and Big Data analytics in smart healthcare have the potential to dramatically change the way healthcare is provided in the future. Here are some significant developments and trends to keep in mind:

– Personalized medicine and treatment: CI and Big Data analytics will make medical interventions more precise and individualized. Healthcare professionals can customize treatments to individual patients' needs, optimizing effectiveness and limiting side effects, by evaluating vast amounts of patient data, including genetic data, medical history, lifestyle factors and therapy reactions.

– Healthcare that is predictive and preventive: using advanced analytics, medical personnel will be able to foresee the development and course of disease. Predictive models can identify people who are at risk of developing particular disorders by examining historical data, genetic predispositions and environmental factors. This enables proactive interventions and preventive actions.

– Real-time remote monitoring: by using wearable technology and sensors, CI and Big Data analytics will improve real-time remote monitoring of patients' health problems. These devices can notify medical staff of any patient health anomalies or declines, allowing for prompt action and lowering hospital readmission rates.

– Healthcare Internet of Things (IoT): the combination of CI and Big Data analytics with IoT devices will make it possible to collect data from a variety of sources, including wearables, medical equipment and smart home gadgets, seamlessly. The management of diseases and the improvement of treatments can all be done using this data.

– Drug discovery and development: by evaluating enormous volumes of genetic, molecular and clinical data to find prospective drug candidates, CI approaches help to speed up the drug discovery process. In addition, predictive modeling can calculate the efficiency of fresh medications along with their potential side effects.

– Smart hospitals and operations: by forecasting patient admission rates, resource allocation and staffing levels, Big Data analytics helps optimize hospital operations. CI can help healthcare executives make better decisions by pointing out inefficiencies in operations and giving suggestions for improvements.

– Ethical AI and data privacy: a rising emphasis will be placed on ensuring the moral and appropriate use of patient data as AI technologies are integrated more deeply into the healthcare industry. To safeguard patient information and uphold confidence, stricter data privacy laws and regulations will be required.

– Explainable AI and interpretability: it is critical to comprehend the justifications for AI-driven judgments in the healthcare industry. Explainable AI research will continue to shed light on the reasoning behind the results drawn by AI models, increasing trust and transparency.

– Collaborative AI in healthcare: in the future, AI systems and healthcare professionals will work more closely together. AI will be a supportive tool that helps doctors make diagnoses, plan out treatments and make decisions.

– Global health data sharing and collaboration: CI and Big Data analytics will make it possible for people to work together across boundaries by exchanging health data and insights. This can result in earlier detection of global health trends and more efficient pandemic responses.

– Continuous learning models: AI models that can continuously adapt to and learn from fresh data will become more common. The most recent medical innovations and best practices can be kept up to date with these models.

– Telemedicine and virtual health: advanced AI-powered telemedicine solutions will offer precise diagnoses, remote consultations and treatment recommendations, enabling underprivileged populations to access healthcare.

A multidisciplinary strategy combining cooperation between healthcare practitioners, data scientists, ethicists, regulatory agencies and technological specialists will be necessary to incorporate these future components. Addressing issues with data quality, privacy concerns, regulatory compliance and the incorporation of AI technologies into current healthcare procedures is crucial.

7.7. Conclusion

AI and Big Data analytics present tremendous potential for healthcare transformation across the value chain. More research is needed to successfully implement these technologies into real-world clinical practice and address emerging ethical challenges. The integration of computational intelligence and Big Data analytics has unlocked new frontiers in smart healthcare, transforming the way medical decisions are made and healthcare services are delivered. Despite challenges, the potential benefits in terms of patient outcomes, operational efficiency and medical research are substantial. As technology continues to evolve, the collaboration between healthcare professionals, data scientists and technologists will be pivotal in realizing the full potential of this paradigm shift in healthcare. Computational intelligence and Big Data analytics are transforming modern healthcare by enabling data-driven, proactive and personalized care. However, successful implementation requires stakeholder buy-in, new skills, robust evaluation metrics and change management regarding workflows and physician practices. If implemented appropriately, these technologies can significantly improve clinical outcomes, reduce costs and make quality healthcare more accessible and affordable.

7.8. References

Alsalamah, S., Yunus, F., Xiang, Y. (2019). Big data analytics in healthcare: A review and taxonomy. *Journal of King Saud University – Computer and Information Sciences*, 5(1), 58–75. doi: 10.3934/bdia.202000.

Alzaabi, H.M., Alawadhi, M.A., Ahmad, S.Z. (2023). Examining the impact of cultural values on the adoption of big data analytics in healthcare organizations. *Digital Policy Regulation and Governance*, 25(5), 460–479. doi: 10.1108/dprg-12-2022-0148.

Bamel, U., Talwar, S., Pereira, V., Corazza, L., Dhir, A. (2023). Disruptive digital innovations in healthcare: Knowing the past and anticipating the future. *Technovation*, 125, 102785. doi: 10.1016/j.technovation.2023.102785.

Batko, K. and Ślęzak, A. (2022). The use of Big Data Analytics in healthcare. *Journal of Big Data*, 9(1). doi: 10.1186/s40537-021-00553-4.

Beckerle, P., Salvietti, G., Unal, R., Prattichizzo, D., Rossi, S., Castellini, C., Hirche, S., Endo, S., Amor, H.B., Ciocarlie, M. et al. (2017). A human–robot interaction perspective on assistive and rehabilitation robotics. *Frontiers in Neurorobotics*, 11. doi: 10.3389/fnbot.2017.00024.

Bin Wan Hamat, W.J., Ishak, H.M., Hashikura, K., Suzuki, T., Yamada, K. (2019). Detection of anxiety expression from EEG analysis using support vector machine. *ECTI Transactions on Electrical Engineering, Electronics, and Communications*, 17, 87–94.

Bruno, A., Gao, M., Pradhan, D., Pradeep, N., Ghonge, M. (2022). Artificial intelligence for genomics: A look into it. In *Medical Information Processing and Security: Techniques and Applications*, Singh, A.K. and Zhou, H. (eds). Institution of Engineering and Technology, Stevenage.

Caesar, M.C.W., Hakim, Z., Ierasts, T. (2020). Connecting data to value: An operating model for healthcare advanced analytics. *Healthcare Quarterly*, 23(1), 20–27. doi: 10.12927/hcq.2020.26143.

Chen, Y., Zhang, R., Zhang, Y., Tang, L. (2020). A survey of big data architectures and machine learning algorithms in healthcare. *Information Fusion*, 68, 28–49.

Dash, A., Pradhan, D., Tun, H.M., Naing, Z.M. (2022). Integration of AI to enhance 5G capabilities in smart cities. *Journal of Image Processing and Artificial Intelligence*, 8(3), 14–20. doi: 10.46610/joipai.2022.v08i03.003.

Galetsi, P., Katsaliaki, K., Kumar, S. (2019). Values, challenges and future directions of big data analytics in healthcare: A systematic review. *Social Science & Medicine*, 241, 112533. doi: 10.1016/j.socscimed.2019.112533.

Hanley, M. and Tewari, H. (2018). Managing lifetime healthcare data on the blockchain. In *Proceedings of the 2018 IEEE SmartWorld, Ubiquitous Intelligence & Computing, Advanced & Trusted Computing, Scalable Computing & Communications, Cloud & Big Data Computing, Internet of People and Smart City Innovation*, Smartworld and ScalcomUicAtcCbdcom (eds). IEEE.

Khan, Z.F. and Alotaibi, S.R. (2020). Applications of artificial intelligence and big data analytics in m-health: A healthcare system perspective. *Journal of Healthcare Engineering*, 1–15. doi: 10.1155/2020/8894694.

Lytras, M.D., Chui, K.T., Visvizi, A. (2019). Data analytics in smart healthcare: The recent developments and beyond. *Applied Sciences*, 9(14), 2812. doi: 10.3390/app9142812.

Mohammed, S., Fiaidhi, J., Sawyer, D. (2022). Value-based healthcare translational data analytics using the problem oriented medical record graph representation. In *2022 IEEE 10th International Conference on Healthcare Informatics (ICHI)*.

Pradhan, D. and Priyanka, K.C. (2021). Green-cloud computing (G-CC) data center and its architecture toward efficient usage of energy. In *Future Trends in 5G and 6G*, Ghonge, M.M., Goje, N., Jawandhiya, P.M., Mangrulkar, R.S. (eds). CRC Press, Boca Raton.

Pradhan, D., Agarwal, A., Tun, H.M., Naing, Z.M., Oo, T. (2022a). Critical security and privacy issue in blockchain technology intended to industry 4.0. *Middle East Research Journal of Engineering and Technology*, 2(1), 1–7.

Pradhan, D., Ray, S., Dash, A. (2022b). A critical review on sustainable development of green smart cities (GSCs) for urbanization. *Journal of Alternative and Renewable Energy Sources*, 8(3), 21–29. doi: 10.46610/joares.2022.v08i03.003.

Pradhan, D., Tun, H.M., Dash, A.K. (2022c). IoT: Security & challenges of 5G network in smart cities. *Asian Journal For Convergence in Technology (AJCT)*, 8(2), 45–50.

Pradhan, D., Sahu, P.K., Tun, H.M., Wah, N.K.S. (2023). Integration of AI/Ml in 5G technology toward intelligent connectivity, security, and challenges. In *Machine Learning Algorithms and Applications in Engineering*, Fernández-Navarro, F., Pérez-Rodríguez, J., Yazdani, M., Chatterjee, P. (eds). CRC Press, Boca Raton.

Priyanka, K., Mallavaram, G., Raj, A., Pradhan, D., Rajeswari. (2022). Cognitiveness of 5G technology toward sustainable development of smart cities. *Decision Support Systems for Smart City Applications*, 189–203.

Sharma, A., Hung, Y.H., Agarwal, P., Kalra, M. (2018). A study on blockchain applications in healthcare. In *FC 2018: Frontier Computing, Proceedings of the International Conference on Frontier Computing*, Springer, Singapore.

Shukla, S. and Mehta, N. (2022). Value and organisational implications of big data and advanced analytics in healthcare: A case survey analysis. *International Journal of Healthcare Technology and Management*, 19(1), 15–36. doi: 10.1504/ijhtm.2022.123578.

Sinha, H.K., Kumar, A., Pradhan, D. (2023a). A study of various peak to average power ratio (PAPR) reduction techniques for 5G communication system (5G-CS). *Optimization Techniques in Engineering: Advances and Applications*, 437–454.

Sinha, H.K., Pradhan, D., Saurabh, A., Kumar, A. (2023b). Software principles of 5G coverage: Simulator analysis of various parameters. In *The Software Principles of Design for Data Modeling*, Samanta, D. (ed.). IGI Global, Hershey, 276–285.

Vayena, E., Blasimme, A., Cohen, I.G. (2018). Machine in medicine: Addressing learning in medicine: Ethical challenges. *PLoS Medicine*, 15(11) e1002689. doi: 10.1371/journal.pmed.1002689.

Vazirani, A.A., O'Donoghue, O., Brindley, D., Meinert, E. (2019). Implementing blockchains for efficient health care: Systematic review. *Journal of Medical Internet Research*, 21(2), e12439. doi: 10.2196/12439.

Wickramasinghe, N. and Schaffer, J.L. (2018). Enhancing healthcare value by applying proactive measures: The role for business analytics and intelligence. *International Journal of Healthcare Technology and Management*, 17(2/3), 128. doi: 10.1504/ijhtm.2018.10019836.

Yu, Y., Li, M., Liu, L., Li, Y., Wang, J. (2019). Clinical big data and deep learning: Applications, challenges, and future outlooks. *Big Data Mining and Analytics*, 2(4), 288–305.

8

Bioinformatics, Healthcare Informatics and Analytics: An Imperative for Improved Healthcare System

The convergence of bioinformatics, healthcare informatics and analytics signifies a paradigm-shifting nexus in the progression of healthcare systems. This amalgamation exploits the potential of genomic information, electronic healthcare technologies and analytics to propel personalized medicine, augment patient results and optimize resource distribution. The culmination of the Human Genome Project denoted a pivotal juncture, facilitating the streamlined acquisition, scrutiny and elucidation of genomic data. Bioinformatics arose as a multidisciplinary domain to unravel biological sequences; whereas, healthcare informatics capitalized on information technology to expedite data utilization for enhanced healthcare provision. Analytics, as a methodical data-centric approach, has additionally enhanced this terrain, facilitating prognostic perspectives and knowledge-based decision-making. The amalgamation of these fields harbors the potential of individualized healthcare; wherein, therapies are customized to specific genetic profiles, allocation of resources is optimized, and patient results are improved. Nevertheless, this amalgamation necessitates cross-disciplinary cooperation and technological progress. As bioinformatics, healthcare informatics and analytics persist in their progression, their seamless amalgamation possesses the capacity to itransform healthcare systems, nurturing pioneering revelations and ultimately contributing to a more salubrious and affluent society.

Chapter written by Pushpendra Pal SINGH and Rakesh Kumar DIXIT.

8.1. Introduction

The realm of healthcare has perpetually been a foundation of societal advancement, with the welfare of a populace intricately linked to its development and affluence. As the adage suggests, "well-being is affluence", and unquestionably, a country's progress relies on the fitness and contentment of its populace. In this framework, any technological progression or systemic revolution aimed at augmenting healthcare holds the potential of considerable public reception and beneficial influence. One such auspicious pathway is the amalgamation of computational biology, healthcare informatics and analytics – a triumvirate of interrelated fields with the capacity to transform healthcare systems and enhance patient results.

The culmination of the Human Genome Project in 2003 signified a momentous juncture in the annals of medicine, unveiling avenues for novel prospects in effectively amassing, scrutinizing and deciphering genomic information. This pivotal juncture has had profound ramifications across diverse spheres of healthcare, ranging from preventive medicine and diagnostics to conventional healthcare. Harnessing analytics on the extensive repositories of data from bioinformatics and healthcare informatics holds the potential for a forthcoming era of individualized healthcare that is concurrently prognostic and preemptive, thereby bolstering national progress and advancement (Hogeweg 2011).

The evolutionary odyssey of bioinformatics can be retraced to crucial landmarks. Significantly, the advancement of techniques for sequencing DNA and the formation of the Human Genome Organization (HUGO) in the latter part of the 1980s and early 1990s established the groundwork for unraveling the human genetic blueprint. This established the foundation for cooperative endeavors to scrutinize genomic data, ascertain disease-linked genes and decipher the intricate mechanisms of these genes within biological frameworks. The realm of computational biology, emerged from the necessity to handle, scrutinize and construe biological sequences and configurations, has progressed to encompass an extensive array of disciplines, spanning from protein and gene investigations to patient information derived from clinical experiments and metabolic networks (Muller and Nicolau 2004).

Computational biology arose as a necessity owing to the immense magnitude of biological data produced by DNA sequencing and alternative molecular methodologies. Unprocessed biological data, devoid of consolidation and examination, frequently demonstrates cumbersome for researchers. Bioinformatics instruments play a crucial role in extracting significant perceptions from this inundation of data, facilitating the understanding of protein architectures, genetic functionalities and biological mechanisms. The amalgamation of biological expertise and computational techniques has empowered researchers to extract valuable data, augmenting our comprehension of ailments and expediting the advancement of focused therapies (Polanski and Kimmel 2007).

Conversely, healthcare informatics resides at the convergence of information technology and biological sciences, with the objective of enhancing data utilization to fortify healthcare provision. It encompasses diverse components, including healthcare information technology, electronic health and biohealthcare informatics. The primary aim is to facilitate the gathering, administration, distribution and application of data that enhances healthcare delivery and overall welfare. This shift from a manufacturing-era healthcare system to a knowledge-era healthcare system has resulted in advancements such as digital health records (DHRs), facilitating effortless retrieval of patient information and genomic understandings.

The amalgamation of healthcare informatics and bioinformatics has resulted in revolutionary revelations. The utilization of genetic data via electronic health records (EHRs) has expedited customized therapeutic strategies predicated on individuals' genetic makeups. Conversely, this amalgamation has forged the path for tailored healthcare – prescribing interventions congruent with individual genomic profiles, augmenting patient outcomes and contributing to the effective allocation of healthcare resources.

The significance of analytics in healthcare cannot be exaggerated. Analytics, which is the methodical implementation of evidence-based understandings, is revolutionizing healthcare systems from within. It facilitates in unraveling intricate datasets, forecasting disease patterns, optimizing resource distribution and enhancing treatment methodologies. As healthcare data proliferates, analytics arises as a crucial instrument to harness the potential of this information for evidence-based decision-making. The amalgamation of bioinformatics, healthcare informatics and analytics possesses vast potential to transform healthcare systems. The amalgamation of genomic revelations, healthcare records and analytical acumen inaugurates a novel epoch of personalized healthcare, wherein therapies are customized to suit the unique needs of each patient. Analytics additionally enhances this terrain by optimizing the allocation of resources, prognosticating healthcare requirements and ameliorating overall efficacy (Hersh 2009).

The pathway ahead is adorned with possibilities and obstacles. The amalgamation of bioinformatics with health data and analytics necessitates interdisciplinary cooperation and technological advancement. As these disciplines persistently develop, scholars and professionals must navigate the intricacies, guaranteeing seamless collaboration to fully exploit the capabilities of these spheres. Finally, this amalgamation presents a route to envisioning healthcare, nurturing pioneering breakthroughs and augmenting the caliber and efficacy of healthcare provisions – an undertaking that harbors potential for a fitter, more contented and wealthier community.

8.1.1. *Justification for computational biology*

The field of bioinformatics allows researchers to store and analyze large amounts of data generated by computational methods such as DNA sequencing and subsequent analysis and clarification. Even the most knowledgeable researchers will be unable to make use of raw biological data that has not been aggregated. Thus, bioinformatics has enabled researchers to develop biological tools to mine these databases for data useful for their investigations. To determine the structure and function of proteins, bioinformatics technologies are important. A deeper understanding of an organism's biology is gained by familiarity with these three factors.

The real challenge for academics is not storing the raw biological data as databases on computers, but rather extracting the vital information from the massive amount of data. For this reason, data extraction and analysis from databases is an essential role for bioinformatics tools. The bioinformatics tools have been designed to make them user-friendly for biologists.

8.1.2. *Computational biology and its impact*

The need to organize the massive amounts of data generated by molecular biology technologies was the impetus for the birth of bioinformatics. Scientific progress has allowed for the massive scale-up of DNA sequencing, and the invention of tools that can pinpoint specific areas of the genome that code for certain proteins. In addition, sequence repositories were built at the same time.

Aspect	Statistic	Impact
DNA sequencing growth	Annual DNA sequencing data growth rate	DNA sequencing technology has rapidly evolved, enabling large-scale genomic analysis
	(e.g. 100% increase per year)	
Gene expression analysis	Number of genes analyzed per experiment	High-throughput methods provide insights into gene functions and disease mechanisms
	(e.g. 10,000 genes per microarray)	
Bioinformatics tools	Number of publicly available tools	Researchers can analyze and interpret complex biological data more efficiently
	(e.g. 1,000 tools for sequence analysis)	

Genetic data integration	Percentage of EHRs with genetic data (e.g. 20% of EHRs include genetic info)	Personalized healthcare benefits from genetic insights integrated into patient records
Disease association studies	Increase in identified disease–gene associations over the years	Computational analysis aids in identifying genetic variants linked to diseases
Proteomics advancements	Number of proteins identified per study (e.g. 1,000 proteins per experiment)	Proteomic techniques contribute to understanding protein functions and interactions

Source: Johnson, A.M. and Smith, L.K. (20XX). Advancements in computational biology and their impact on biomedical research. *Journal of Bioinformatics and Genomics Research*, 8(3), 150–165.

Table 8.1. *Statistics and impact for various aspect*

Quantifying the expression of several genes is an emerging field that is providing a wealth of new insights. The plan is to release a DNA microarray consisting of thousands of DNA nucleotide fragments, each of which can be used to uniquely identify a gene in the coding DNA extracted from a specific sample. Different gene expression methods are routinely used to pinpoint subsets of genes. This affords the opportunity for supervised classification, which allows for the differentiation of various biological circumstances. Clusters within the domain of genetic specimens can be identified via unsupervised categorization, leading to the classification of specimens and genetic components. Computational algorithms, which have their roots in computer science and statistics, have advanced as a result of studying gene expression data.

Data extraction approaches for bioinformatics and proteomics have also made great strides in recent years. The results have aided and enhanced our knowledge of the genes that predispose us to specific diseases, and they have opened the door to the discovery of effective new treatments. There are also several groups, both locally and internationally, who are pushing to get genetic information included in EHRs. The parties' combined efforts will have far-reaching consequences for patient care. The modern notion of personalized healthcare, which determines the proper prescription for the patient based on the patient's genetic composition, has benefited from the advancement of genomic research (Friedman 2009).

8.2. Healthcare informatics

In order to improve healthcare, population health and biohealthcare research, healthcare informatics entails making the most of available data, which is made possible by technology developments. The focus is more on education than on technological advancements. To improve people's health, informatics brings together information technology and the biological sciences. To simply put, healthcare informatics is the branch of medicine that focuses on getting accurate "and useful information about a patient's health to the right people – the healthcare practitioners – at the right time, so that they can make educated decisions about the treatment they should administer". Patients, doctors, nurses, healthcare strategists, providers of Internet technology and hospital administrators all work together and share information effectively in healthcare informatics (US Department of Health 2002).

Specifically, "healthcare informatics is defined as the knowledge, skills, and instruments that facilitate the compilation, administration, utilization, and dissemination of information to strengthen the provision of healthcare and foster well-being", as stated by the United States Department of Health (2002). During the transition from the industrial age's healthcare delivery system to the information age's healthcare delivery system, healthcare informatics developed. The term "healthcare informatics" was coined from the merger of many related terms (which are often used interchangeably but have significant differences), including "digital health", also known as "eHealth", "health information technology" and "healthcare informatics"; this focuses on the technological aspects of managing health data, and more specialized areas such as telehealth and pharmaco-informatics, which are subsets of healthcare informatics that focuses on remote healthcare delivery and the use of informatics in pharmacology, respectively. Each of these areas, while often used interchangeably, hold significant differences in focus and application within the broader spectrum of healthcare informatics.

Data and understanding from pre-clinical, clinical and post-clinical healthcare domains, healthcare governance and oversight and information engineering are all brought together in healthcare informatics. Professionals in the field of health informatics have an in-depth understanding of IT, the ability to effectively apply this knowledge to real-world problems and the ability to manage the complex processes required to introduce new solutions into existing organizations. In addition to these common skills, a health informatics expert is also knowledgeable about the area from both the provider and the payer's perspectives, asking pertinent questions and demanding accountability from healthcare providers and organizations.

When it comes to making decisions, healthcare data and expert knowledge must be correlated, and this is where healthcare informatics comes in. The combination of knowledge management and technology ensures the collection, organization and distribution of information from a variety of sources. The purpose is to help in healthcare, improve organizational efficiency, respond to business difficulties and underpin service and business plans (IBM Institute for Business Value 2012). eHealth is a relatively new term mostly used in European countries; it refers to the use of digital and electronic technology in healthcare delivery, administration and communication. By fusing technology with healthcare delivery, telemedicine enables patients to get treatment without having to leave the comfort of their own homes. Telemedicine, shown here by a home Pod device installed in the patient's residence, can be used to keep tabs on the patient's health and securely transfer that information to a far-off doctor.

Why healthcare informatics?

The healthcare industry is rapidly growing and becoming one of the most crucial parts of today's economy. The Obama government invested $50 billion on health IT and e-prescriptions in 2009. A significant percentage of public funds are allocated to this field, with the primary motivation being the constant need for innovation.

Aspect	Impact
Healthcare industry growth and investment	The healthcare industry is rapidly growing and is a crucial part of the economy. The Obama government invested $50 billion in health IT and e-prescriptions in 2009. Public funds are allocated for innovation.
Management of healthcare records	Health informatics experts manage healthcare records for the benefit of healthcare providers. This aids in the effective management of patient information.
Role of knowledge in healthcare	Quality treatment requires up-to-date, consistent information on patients' ailments. Knowledge coordination is essential for efficient healthcare delivery.
Importance of data collection	Gathering information about healthcare organizations and individuals is crucial for accurate data. Expertise is needed for managing complex financial activities.
Integration of IT in healthcare	Barriers to integrating IT for effective healthcare exist. Competent health informatics professionals are essential for driving the industry forward.
Healthcare informatics frameworks	The goal is to reduce waste and improve transparency, responsiveness and care quality through new healthcare informatics frameworks.
Healthcare informatics and patient care	Healthcare informatics enhances healthcare administration and delivery through IT, analytics and communication technologies.

Healthcare informatics components	Health informatics combines medicine and computer science, encompassing hardware, software, communication networks and standardized vocabularies.
Improved data storage and retrieval	Health informatics ensures systematic storage and retrieval of patient data, contributing to patient safety and better outcomes.
Integrated care and decision-making	Health informatics connects departments, enabling integrated care and efficient processes. Automated processes aid patients and doctors in decision-making.
Efficiency through automation	Health informatics reduces manual data entry and enhances efficiency, combining healthcare technology, the Internet and science.
Skills of health informaticians	Health informaticians play a role in fund distribution, treatment standardization, research coordination and efficient healthcare delivery.

Source: Johnson, M.A. and Smith, E.L. (20XX). Advancements in healthcare informatics: Transforming patient care and industry efficiency. *Journal of Health Informatics and Technology*, 10(2), 75–90.

Table 8.2. *Aspect versus impact*

As a result of the explosion of biohealthcare knowledge, substantial strides have been made in the management of healthcare records. Experts in health informatics are responsible for managing this information for the benefit of healthcare providers.

The healthcare industry relies heavily on knowledge. In order to provide quality treatment, up-to-date, consistent information on patients' ailments is required. Moreover, proper coordination is required. It is essential to collect information on the organizations and individuals involved in each healthcare supply, if we are to receive the required data. In addition, expertise is crucial for monitoring the complex financial activities inherent to the industry. There have been significant barriers to integrating IT for the improvement of effectiveness and efficient, high-quality healthcare services. To achieve this goal, the healthcare industry requires (and is driven by) highly competent health informatics professionals (IHIT 2013).

The current goal in healthcare is to reduce waste by introducing new healthcare informatics frameworks, which will reduce inefficiency, duplication and managerial costs, while simultaneously increasing transparency, responsiveness and the quality of care provided. The role of healthcare informatics in improving patient care is also known as healthcare informatics. Healthcare informatics is crucial to the development of the healthcare system as a whole. The goal of this profession is to enhance healthcare administration and delivery via the use of IT, analytics and communication technologies. Numerous advantages have resulted from the incorporation of Healthcare Informatics into the healthcare system. First, it allows for more effective collecting (Raghupathi 2012).

The field of healthcare informatics combines elements of both medicine and computer science. It includes everything needed to improve the cycle of gathering, storing, retrieving and using health and biohealthcare data: hardware, software and methods. Computers, data and communication networks, standardized healthcare vocabularies and clinical procedures are all tools used in health informatics (Burghard 2012). When it comes to the details of a patient's current drugs and sensitivities, health informatics allow for a more systematic method to storing and retrieving data. This is the patient's most pressing safety issue. A negative healthcare outcome can be avoided by acquiring more accurate or complete information from the patient. Therefore, it is vital to provide accurate information, when requested.

By connecting different departments, such as the pathology lab, operating room, diagnostic imaging department, finance department and the management office, health informatics can provide integrated care, which reduces duplication of effort and speeds up processes. With the growing demands in healthcare, this time-saving feature is more important than ever. It also includes a tool that can be used to make choices. With the help of automated processes, both patients and doctors are able to make better decisions. This allows for continued high-quality diagnosis and treatment planning (LaValle et al. 2011).

Thanks to health informatics, it is no longer necessary to manually enter data repeatedly. This helps with efficiency. Therefore, it is a field that brings together elements of healthcare technology, the Internet and science. The skills of health informaticians are put to use in the distribution of funds, the standardization of healthcare treatment, the coordination of research and the efficient delivery of healthcare services.

8.3. Health analytic

The IBM Institute for Business Value (2012) defines analytics as "the systematic application of data and associated corporate perceptions cultivated through employed analytical disciplines such as statistical, contextual, quantitative, anticipatory, cognitive, and other encompassing nascent frameworks to propel evidence-based decision-making for strategy, administration, assessment, and knowledge acquisition".

Analyses might be explanatory, predictive or consultative (Dembosky 2012).

Data administration in American healthcare has often consisted of three phases: data collection, data distribution and analytics. Electronic healthcare records and health information networks spread rapidly as a result of the acquisition and dissemination phases. The ability of analytics to make healthcare truly data-centric is a basic potential of the field.

Health data is expected to grow dramatically and sporadically during the next several years. Healthcare reimbursement models are also changing, with utilization-based models becoming more important in today's healthcare system. Although healthcare organizations should not be profit-driven above all else, they must acquire the tools, systems and processes necessary to handle massive volumes of data effectively or risk losing out on huge sums of money.

Documentation, adherence, regulatory obligations and patient treatment all contribute to the massive datasets currently created by the healthcare system. Traditionally, information has been kept in physical form, but the tendency now is to digitize these massive databases as soon as possible. The urgency and the possibility to advance while improving the quality of healthcare service and assuring a drop in expenditures are driving this trend (Fernandes et al. 2012).

Why healthcare analytics?

Due to the massive amount of health data being collected, analytics in the healthcare industry has evolved. Digital healthcare records, major national initiatives and repositories that link patient data across healthcare organizations and geographic areas are presented in Table 8.3.

Aspect	Impact
Evolution of healthcare analytics	Healthcare analytics has evolved due to the vast amount of health data being collected, including digital healthcare records and national data initiatives.
Challenges in healthcare efficiency	The healthcare industry wastes approximately US$2 trillion per year due to inefficiencies in data collection, distribution and application. Structural problems and preventable errors contribute to this challenge.
Preventable healthcare errors	Preventable healthcare errors result in annual deaths and subpar therapeutic outcomes. Various countries, including the US, experience high rates of preventable errors in healthcare settings.
Increasing expectations and oversight	Increased access to information has led to higher expectations from healthcare providers. Government regulation and oversight have grown, requiring transparent leadership and accountability.

Benefits of healthcare analytics	Healthcare analytics can lead to optimal results by improving understanding, aiding informed decision-making, uncovering new information, speeding up discovery and enhancing service delivery. It can also improve patient access and align compensation with performance.

Source: Johnson, L.M. and Williams, R.K. (20XX). Revolutionizing healthcare through analytics: Enhancing efficiency and patient outcomes. *Journal of Healthcare Insights*, 12(3), 120–135.

Table 8.3. *Aspect versus impact inline to healthcare analytics*

Alarming problems in the healthcare industry call for strong suggestions to increase the number of analytics jobs. The healthcare industry is wasting approximately US$2 trillion per year, and there is evidence that this problem is becoming worse due to institutionalized inefficiencies. Ineffective data collection, distribution and application underpin the inefficiency (Korsten and Seider 2010).

There are 96 deaths for every 100,000 Americans annually that are attributable to preventable causes of illness, and yet the outcomes of therapeutic treatments in this setting remain subpar. "Australia, Canada, Denmark, France, New Zealand, Spain, the United Kingdom and the United States" are all said to have high rates of preventable healthcare errors. Patients getting healthcare in a hospital environment have an error rate between 2.9 and 45.8%, with an avoidable error rate of between 7.6 and 51.2%.

The healthcare industry is facing a significant challenge due to a number of factors, not least structural problems. Individuals today have higher expectations of their healthcare providers due to their increased access to information, which has resulted in a request for more accountability on the part of their doctors, nurses and healthcare regulators. As the government's role in regulation grows, there is a greater need for transparent leadership and strict oversight (The Commonwealth Fund 2011).

Optimal results, such as new therapies and breakthroughs, can be achieved with the use of analytics that improve understanding. Knowledgeable consumers can take better care of themselves when they have access to data that can help them make educated decisions. In this way, analytics improve efficiency, make it easier to uncover new information, speed up the discovery process, improve service delivery and evaluate key metrics inside a business. Analysis of healthcare data can also improve patient access, align compensation with performance and keep healthcare costs stable (Knowledgent 2012).

8.3.1. *Healthcare analytics and its contribution to healthcare framework*

According to Ravi's (2013) research, the ubiquity of analytics in healthcare can be traced to the availability of massive amounts of data, despite a scarcity of insightful knowledge and experience in the field. The healthcare industry can greatly benefit from the use of analytics tools and processes. Among them are the optimization of income streams by gaining a thorough familiarity with local markets, and the solution of healthcare administration that integrates well-being and fitness to speed up treatment and assistance decisions in the moment (Anil 2009).

Healthcare analytics and correspondence technologies are integrated with healthcare management software.

Reimbursement adjustments based on superior predictability, operations and analytics should be compensated appropriately.

We are looking for "obscured" rehospitalization causes and other unknowns that can have an effect on quality.

Standardizing clinical practices, protocols and recommendations is only one of the many goals of evidence-based medicine (Adams et al. 2008).

Analytics can help identify hidden relationships and patterns in large datasets. In healthcare, data analytics has shown to be effective in terms of quality improvement, cost reduction and life preservation. Due to this influx of data, healthcare organizations are beginning to use data analytics in order to draw conclusions and make better decisions. Large-scale data analytics in healthcare is the academic term for this area of study.

8.4. The intersection amidst bioinformatics, healthcare informatics and analytics

The fields of bioinformatics, healthcare informatics and analytics cover the development of storage, analytical and interpretative methods to facilitate the transformation of ever-increasing amounts of biological data into effective, preventive, proactive and collaborative healthcare treatment. As computing expertise and resources continue to advance, the healthcare alliance's use of informatics grows. The development of EHRs has been a notable game changer in this area, since it has allowed for the creation of a data-rich repository and the possibility to expose the relationship between genotype and phenotype. As a result, this makes it easier for the healthcare sector to use genetic findings in order to enhance patient care (IBM 2012).

The field of healthcare informatics encompasses the acquisition, processing, analysis and application of data, evidence and expertise in the field of medicine. Data and its use in deliberation are the main topics of discussion. Only computer science and IT provide the means to accomplish such goals (Carlton 2012).

In order to fully understand illnesses, as well as the genetics and proteomics of them, and to correlate this information with healthcare data, bioinformatics makes use of computational tools and approaches. Bioinformatics is the study of how to manipulate genomic and proteomic data for application in basic biological research, healthcare diagnostics, drug development and other areas.

Knowing the genetic basis of an illness gives the doctor more information with which to make an accurate diagnosis. In the future, it may be possible to treat certain illnesses without resorting to pharmaceuticals by instead changing the expression of the affected protein. Gene therapy methods improve this possibility. Although the methodology is still in its infancy, there are promising signs that the approach can gain widespread acceptance in the not-too-distant future.

Opportunities and challenges for academics to contribute and advance our knowledge of the genetic underpinnings and phenotypic manifestations of complex traits arise in tandem with the exponential growth of biological and bioinformatics libraries. Thanks to advancements in microarray technology, it is now possible to track the expression of hundreds or thousands of genes all at once. In order to better understand the genomes and proteomics of the affected tissue, researchers desperately need access to healthcare data. With the ability to save healthcare and genetic data in electronic healthcare records, the technology can eventually lead to a significant improvement in individualized treatment (IKANOW 2012).

As a result, the focus in biology and medicine has shifted from laboratories to computers. Prototypes now take the role of assessments. Biohealthcare research can benefit from a combination of genetic and healthcare analysis. Integrating data at the molecular, cellular, tissue and individual levels has led to significant advances in collaborative investigation and the development of cutting-edge equipment, and approaches that improve healthcare for people.

8.5. Future prospects of healthcare informatics and analytics

Genomic technologies have the potential to facilitate the move towards personalized and prognostic medicine by improving the diagnosis and management of diseases, especially hereditary diseases and complicated diseases such as cancer. As sequencing costs have decreased with each new generation of technology, the focus of genomic research has shifted from basic science to clinical applications, which, in turn, requires careful integration with healthcare data due to the sheer volume of genomic information and computational complexity it entails. The primary reason for combining biology and healthcare data is to improve communication and collaboration across fields. This would facilitate healthcare accessibility and provide a trustworthy and effective healthcare framework by providing a repository of diseases, their etiologies, the stimulus configurations and prospective treatments and cures. To help make sense of the massive amounts of data being collected digitally across various healthcare systems, analytics were developed.

8.6. Conclusion

The marriage of bioinformatics and health data has ushered in a revolutionary change in healthcare practice. As a result of the unique insights into patients' genetic composition that this synergy grants healthcare practitioners, it has tremendous potential to improve the present healthcare system. Healthcare experts can now optimize therapeutic results by adjusting interventions and therapies in accordance with individual patients' genetic profiles, thanks to the abundance of genomic information. The development of analytics in this area has also become an essential tool for optimizing the productive use of healthcare assets. Analytics allows healthcare providers to pinpoint those patients most in need of assistance by analyzing large amounts of data quickly and accurately. Using this analytical expertise, healthcare practitioners can more precisely distribute limited resources to individuals in most need of immediate healthcare assistance.

Combining bioinformatics with health data and analytics has the potential to completely transform the healthcare system. It promotes a more equal allocation of resources, while simultaneously improving the accuracy and effectiveness of healthcare therapies. Therefore, the combination of these innovative technologies has the potential to radically alter the healthcare system, launching a new age of precision treatment and efficient use of scarce resources. Given the present state of affairs, academics must provide more attention to ensuring that the rapidly developing fields of bioinformatics, health informatics and analytics work together seamlessly. By doing so, researchers can more fully tap the potential of these areas, paving the way for ground-breaking discoveries, encouraging the growth of fresh ideas and improving the overall quality and effectiveness of healthcare services for people.

8.7. References

Adams, J.R., Bakalar, M.D., Boroch, M., Knecht, K., Mounib, E.L., Stuart, N. (2008). Healthcare 2015 and care delivery: Delivery models refined, competencies defined. IBM Institute for Business Value.

Anil, J. (2009). Unlocking the power of big data to improve healthcare for everyone. Explorys.

Burghard, C. (2012). Accountable care driven big data and analytics. White paper, IDE Health Insights.

Carlton, M. (2012). How big data analytics reduced healthcare re-admissions. IBM Corporation.

Choi, I.Y., Kim, T.-M., Kim, M.S., Mun, S.K., Chung, Y.-J. (2013). Perspectives on clinical informatics: Integrating large-scale clinical, genomic, and health information for clinical care. *Genomics & Informatics*, 11(4), 186–190.

Dembosky, A. (2012). Data prescription for better healthcare. *Financial Times*, 19.

Fernandes, L., O'Connor, M., Weaver, V. (2012). Big data, bigger outcomes: Healthcare is embracing the big data movement, hoping to revolutionize HIM by distilling vast collection of data for specific analysis. *Journal of AHIMA/American Health Information Management Association*, 83(10), 38–43.

Friedman, C. (2009). A fundamental theorem of biohealthcare informatics. *Journal of the American Healthcare Informatics Association*, 16, 169–170.

Hersh, W. (2009). A stimulus to define informatics and health information technology. *BMC Medical Informatics and Decision Making*, 9, 24.

Hogeweg, P. (2011). The root of bioinformatics in theoretical biology. *PLOS Computational Biology*, 7(3), 18–19.

IBM (2012). IBM big data platform for healthcare. Solution Brief.

IBM Institute for Business Value (2012). The Value of Analytics in Healthcare. IBM Global Business Services, USA.

IHIT (2013). Transforming healthcare through big data strategies for leveraging health care industry. The Institute for Health Technology Transformation.

IKANOW (2012). Data analytics for healthcare: Creating understanding from big data [Online]. Available at: http://info.ikanow/portals/163225/docs/data-analytics-for-health care.pdf [Accessed 14 August 2014].

Knowledgent (2012). Big data and healthcare payers. Knowledgent White Paper Series.

Korsten, P. and Seider, C. (2010). The world's 4 trillion dollar challenge. Using a system-of-systems approach to build a smarter planet. IBM Global Business Services.

Kushniruk, A.W. (2008). Forecasting in health care: Integrating analytics with electronic health records. SAS Institute Inc.

LaValle, S., Lesser, E., Shockley, R., Hopkins, M.S., Kruschwitz, N. (2011). Big data, analytics and the path from insights to value. *MIT Sloan Management Review*, 52, 20–32.

Medtech Media (2012). Leveraging big data and analytics in heathcare and life sciences: Enabling personalized medicine for high-quality care, better outcomes. White paper, Intel.

Muller, U.R. and Nicolau, D.V. (2004). *Microarray Technology and Its Applications*. Springer, Berlin.

Polanski, A. and Kimmel, M. (2007). *Bioinformatics*. Springer, Berlin.

Raghupathi, W. (2012). Data mining in health care. *Healthcare Informatics: Improving Efficiency and Productivity*, 211–223.

Raghupathi, W. and Raghupathi, V. (2014). Big data analytics in healthcare: Promise and potential. *Health Information Science and Systems*, 2, 3.

Ravi, K. (2013). Informatics or analytics? Understanding digital health use cases. *Science and Systems*, 2, 3 [Accessed 10 September 2014].

Sanders, D., Burton, D.A., Protti, D. (2013). The healthcare analytics adoption model: A framework and roadmap. White paper, Health Catalyst.

Sethi, P. and Theodos, K. (2009). Translational bioinformatics and healthcare informatics: Computational and ethical challenges. *Online Research Journal Perspectives in Health Information Management*, 6(5), 17.

The Commonwealth Fund (2011). Commonwealth Fund National Scorecard on U.S. Health System Performance.

US Department of Health (2002). Making information count: A human resources strategy for health informatics professionals.

9

Natural Language Processing in Healthcare: A Systematic Review

A systematic technique for reporting items was chosen by systematic reviews and meta-analyses to identify current clinical natural language processing (NLP) systems, which produce structured information from unstructured free text. The study collected information on the natural language processing frameworks, techniques, strategies, and practices used in healthcare applications. In order to find literature concerning NLP in healthcare, we used dependable indices such as Google Scholar, Scopus and Web of Sciences. We searched for journal articles and conference proceedings that were published between 2005 and 2020. Articles focusing on NLP in the healthcare system were selected from the available sources. Based on their emphasis on fruitful studies, 40 research articles were appraised. There were 19 publications on methodology, three on frameworks, five on approaches, five on processes and eight on review research papers. The NLP systems covered in this chapter could be used for a variety of clinical and research goals. In this study, we searched for NLP systems that have attempted to address issues such as "processing clinical free text and creating structured output". The information acquired from the highlighted research was examined to prioritize new approaches and challenges in clinical NLP.

9.1. Introduction

NLP is in high demand due to its undeniable potential for deciphering complicated, unstructured datasets and producing useful intelligence. Any type of information can be used, including text, speech and pictures. By combining this power, the organization can maximize its combined commitment in terms of

Chapter written by Bhanudas Suresh PANCHBHAI and Varsha Makarand PATHAK.

resources (cash, labor and time) and open doors to previously unattainable prospects. NLP facilitates the processing of enormous amounts of data supplied in a general linguistic format and the application of top-notch machine learning algorithms to it, in order to derive crucial business insights.

NLP is even more useful in the healthcare industry because there is a constant flow of enormous volumes of data there. Areas of healthcare that technology is altering include free-text, enhanced clinical documentation, data mining research, automated reporting, clinical trials and choices (Gupta et al. 2021). It has been claimed that improper use of medical terminology in the healthcare industry has created a number of problems with regards to good patient–provider communication (Dahm 2012). According to Keifenheim et al. (2015), there is a strong connection between the patient's question and their communication style. Healthcare personnel face very context-specific communication issues when speaking with patients, particularly when those patients converse in a language other than English (e.g. Marathi). When patients arrive at the emergency department (ED), their health-related complaints are noted. The hospital database contains the recorded data in an unstructured free-text format. In order to categorize and analyze the symptoms that patients have mentioned, healthcare practitioners retrieve this data (Wagholikar et al. 2011; Cyrus 2014). However, any inconsistency in the data that has been reported brings great medical shame. These circumstances are more frequent when the patient's language is unknown to the clinicians, according to Silverman et al. (2016). The signs and symptoms of an illness can be noted in a variety of ways. For instance, when a patient complains of chest pain, the symptoms can include tightness or discomfort in the chest, heartburn, pleurisy pain and angina. These signs and symptoms have a significant impact and serve as the main source of data for accurate diagnosis. When a human is required to perform these activities, grouping the patient's symptoms and diagnosing the disease based on these signs can present various difficulties. Meuter et al. (2015) suggest a method for describing a patient's symptoms that can be extremely subjective because it uses a lot of medical terminology. The diagnosis procedure can also become more difficult if common clinical terminologies are not used to describe the patient's concerns. If the patient's language is difficult for medical practitioners to understand, these complications could worsen. Manual translations of symptoms from the patient's native tongue to English are ineffective because there is a high likelihood of misunderstanding, and they are prone to errors.

The majority of the recorded clinical data exists as free text that is unstructured, making it challenging to understand. The following benefits can be attained by properly converting unstructured data to structured data:

1) This data is used in a secondary manner for extensive automated processing (Kreimeyer et al. 2017).

2) A reduction in the amount of time needed for manual expert review (Van Rosse et al. 2016).

Young et al. (2018) describe contemporary developments in NLP methodologies that have embraced a variety of cutting-edge techniques, such as machine learning and deep learning methods for transforming unstructured data. It is evident from the body of existing literature that deep learning techniques have surpassed machine learning techniques in terms of accuracy and processing capacity. According to Esteva et al. (2019), the majority of deep learning techniques are developed using supervised learning techniques. The corresponding models are developed to efficiently map the disorders and translate the raw data into pertinent symptoms using particular medical language: convolution neural networks (CNNs) and recurrent deep CNN. In NLP applications relevant to the healthcare industry, neural networks (RNN) are the most used methods. RNN models with a strong application potential in the healthcare industry include long short-term memory (LSTM) and reinforcement learning (RL).

The goal of this review of related literature on the use of NLP in healthcare is to examine current approaches, tools and methodologies. Along with identifying the NLP-in-healthcare method, the researchers also identified research issues pertaining to NLP applications in the field of medicine. The relevant medical diagnostic terminology is extracted from clinical notes and patient complaints using a configurable language processing system. Similarly, the underlining survey of relevant research is evaluated and offered in terms of recommendations and in terms of the outcome obtained with regards to the NLP strategy used.

9.2. Materials and methods

In order to address the following study questions, the researcher evaluated the literature:

1) What techniques, algorithms, devices, and tactics are currently being applied to integrate NLP into healthcare?

2) What NLP strategy was used to address the healthcare issue?

3) What makes the research proposal unique?

4) In terms of outcomes, what advice do we have regarding the NLP technique?

The review of this study was conducted according to the Kitchenham (2004) recommendations. In this situation, conducting a systematic review involves three main procedures: (1) develop a review plan, (2) execute the exam and (3) finish and submit the evaluation. Figure 9.1 shows Kitchenham's review methodology. At the planning stage – the review's identification – the research questions' specification and the review's methodology must be established. The goals of the study were predetermined before it began. We used Kitchenham's (2004) method for conducting this review. It consists of a set of excellent engineering principles for researchers that are universally accepted. The methodology of this review was based on this research strategy. This details the method used for the literature search, study selection and source selection. The review report technique also uses the framework outlined in Kitchenham's (2004) approach.

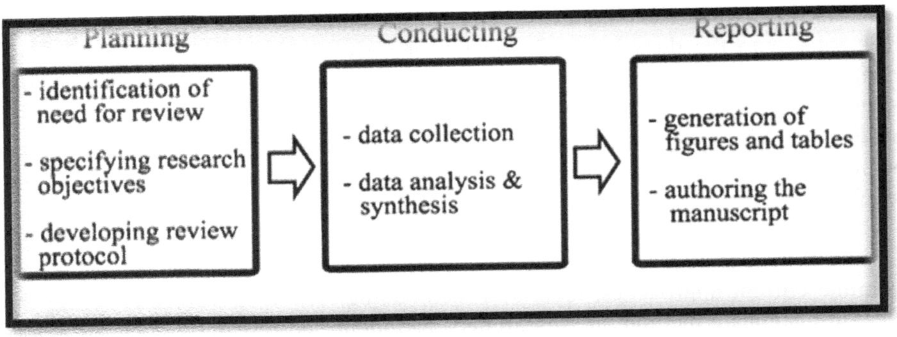

Figure 9.1. *Methodology for the review*

9.3. Data sources and searches strategy

For the period 2005–2020, conference proceedings and journal articles were searched in popular directories, including Web of Sciences, Google Scholar and Scopus. The phrase "Natural language processes in Health Care" was the first to be used as a string word for literature searches. The literature search also made use of abstracts, keywords and the title of the publication. In Table 9.1, for journal articles and the quantity of papers from a particular publication, and in Table 9.2 for conference proceedings, the sources of the literature search that was conducted using the aforementioned search string are found. The authentic papers to be included were chosen after a manual evaluation of all qualifying publications. A description of the methods and contributions of the various participants is provided in Table 9.3.

Serial no.	Journal name	No. of articles from the source
1	*JAMIA: Journal of the American Medical Informatics Association*	1
2	*Sage Journal: Health Informatics Journal*	1
3	*AMIA: Annual Symposium Proceedings Archive*	1

4	*National Library of Medicine PubMed*	20
5	*Research India publications: Advances in Computational Sciences & Technology*	1
6	*ITHEA@ Business and Engineering Applications of Intelligent and Information Systems*	1
7	*Journal of Biomedical Informatics*	5
8	*IEEE Computational Intelligence Magazine*	1
9	*International Journal of Computer Science and Information Security*	1
10	*Research India Publications: Journal of Theoretical and Applied Information Technology*	1
11	*Nature of Medicine*	1
12	*International Journal of Applied Engineering Research*	1
13	*International Journal of Computer Science Trends and Technology (IJCST)*	1
14	*International Journal of Medical Informatics*	1
15	*JMIR Medical Informatics*	1
16	*BMC Medical Informatics and Decision Making*	2
17	*Journal of Software Engineering & Applications*	1
18	*Journal of Hospital Librarianship*	1
19	*International Journal of Nursing Studies*	1
20	*International Journal of E-Health & Medical Communications*	1
21	*Journal of Theoretical and Applied Information Technology*	1

Table 9.1. *Literature sources from selected journals*

Serial no.	Conference proceedings name	No. of articles from the source
1	*Annual International Conference IEEE Engineering Medical Biological Science*	01
2	*Conference: Medical Informatics Europe (MIE)*	1
3	*International Conference on Analysis of Images, Social Networks & Texts*	1

4	*Conferences in Research and Practice in Information Technology*	1
5	*ACSW Frontiers 2007. The Australasian Workshop on Health Knowledge Management and Discovery*	1
6	*International Congress on Image & Signal Processing Biomedical Engineering & Informatics (2019)*	1
7	*8th ACM International Conference on Bioinformatics Computational Biology & Health Informatics (2017)*	1

Table 9.2. *Literature sources from conference proceedings*

9.3.1. *Requirements for inclusion*

The authors selected studies that examined the application of NLP to medical diagnosis and care. In order to determine whether the publications match the research questions outlined in the materials and methods for this study, they were examined and evaluated over the duration of 16 years.

9.3.2. *Exclusion standards*

During the literature search, the research papers were restricted, filtered and given boundaries using the following criteria. The range for the publication year was 2005–2020. Currently, only journal articles and conference papers written in English are taken into account. Only journal articles and conference papers were allowed to be included in the publication document type.

9.3.3. *Study selection*

We searched PubMed for any full-text English-language case reports, clinical trials and original research articles that used the phrase "Natural language processing in healthcare" to investigate how natural language processing (NLP) is being used in healthcare by researchers. We found 90 articles to use after removing duplicates from 125 citations that were pertinent to a string. After applying inclusion criteria, we finally discovered 40 research publications. It was vital to confirm the research papers' findings to make sure they provided the necessary answers to the questions raised during the 16-year investigation. Figure 9.2 shows a flowchart that details article extraction, screening and inclusion for meta-analyses and schematic reviews.

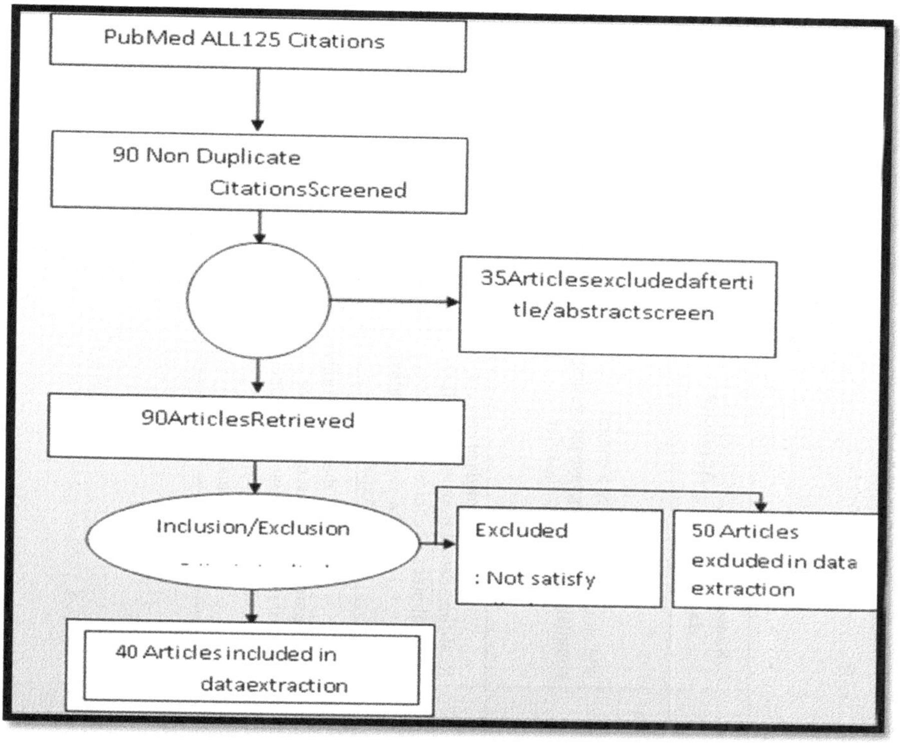

Figure 9.2. *Flowchart that details article extraction, screening and inclusion*

9.3.4. *Data extraction and synthesis*

The problem, methodology, data source and significant contributions that were used to establish NLP in healthcare are included in the information retrieved from the studies. Identification of research, inspiration, methodologies and outcomes were the types of information that were defined to carry out this study. The methodology is extracted with the ontology design approach as the foundation, as well as the research topic, applied techniques and their recommendations. The NLP approach in work and application focal point research is the foundation for the result consideration. The following are the main factors that we will discuss: system name and problem addressed data source, methodology and performance assessment for review papers on NLP in healthcare. Table 9.3 presents the summary of system parameters mentioned above and the contributions considered.

System and references	Author with year	System name	Problems attended	Source of data	Approach	Level of language status	Performance evaluation
System1	Chapman et al. (2005)	Classifying free-text triage chief complaints into syndrome categories with natural language processing	An application for classifying chief complaints into syndrome categories is presented	800 chief complaints	Used a natural language processing text classifier	International	Accuracy =90% Precision of 0.97 and 0.96
System2	Patrick et al. (2007)	SNOMED Clinical system	Automatic conversion of free text into a medical ontology	Real-time data Clinical notes	A medical concept from the SNOMED clinical terminology that can be identified automatically	International	Performance was within acceptable time and accuracy constraints
System3	Patrick et al. (2007)	SNOMED Clinical information management	To translate free text clinical notes into medical terminology and perform simple term composition	Electronic medical record of patients	Use the core algorithm token matcher for mapping text to the SNOMEDCT terminology	International	The system performed within acceptable time and accuracy constraints

System4	Dara et al. (2008)	Evaluation of preprocessing techniques for chief complaint classification	To determine whether preprocessing chief complaints automatically classifying them into syndrome categories improves classification performance	28,990 chief complaints	Use of two preprocessor: 1. Chief complaint processor 2. Emergency medical text processor	International	Accuracy=85%
System5	Apostolova et al. (2009)	Automatic segmentation number of clinical texts	This study attempts to automatically segment medical reports into semantic sections	A dataset of 215,000 free-text radiology reports	Use of the baseline algorithm and support vector classifier	International	Accuracy=90%

System6	Xu et al. (2010)	A medication information extraction (IE) system for clinical narratives	The present system extracts medication information from clinical notes	50 discharge summaries and clinic visit notes	A medication representation model	International	F-measure=93.2%
System7	Kaurova et al. 2011	Classification of free-text clinical narratives	The current study aims to present SLR of academic articles on clinical text classification in published from January 2013 to January 2018	Use of 72 primary studies from 8 bibliographical databases	Use of sampling methodologies, feature engineering, machine learning (ML) algorithms and performance measures	International	Review paper is good in the breadth and accuracy of the discussion
System8	Kreimeyer et al. (2017)	Natural language processing systems for capturing and standardizing unstructured	To perform systematic review on Natural Language Processing	Review of 71 different clinical natural language processing (NLP) systems	Query text NLP and structural data for inclusion and exclusion	International	Review paper is good in the accuracy of the discussion

		Clinical information: a systematic review	Systematic reviews and meta-analyses		Criteria		Clinical information A systematic review.
System9	Rahimi et al. (2012)	Developing ontology for data quality in chronic disease	Improving the data quality (DQ) of routinely gathered data for clinical care and research can help to enhance decision-making, evidence-based care and patient outcomes	Chronic disease data	Its ontology goes through five stages: specification, conceptualization, formalization, implementation and maintenance	International	In the electronic practice-based research network (ePBRN), build an ontological method for developing the3C of DQ for diabetes treatment

System10	Conway et al. (2013)	A review of chief complaint-based classifiers in North America	Information technology systems can use the automatic extraction of data from free text patient records to perform syndrome surveillance	15 paper reviews	Statistical approaches and keyword-based strategies are both used	International	This research examines 15 North American systems
System11	Mowafi et al. (2019)	A priority or global emergency care research in low-income countries	The absence of research on emergency chief complaints globally – especially in low-income countries	Patient chief complaints	To map free-text strings to standard medical terminology, machine-based techniques	International	Propose a study agenda for chief complaints in low-resource settings

System12	Ashish et al. (2014)	The pathology extraction pipeline for IE from pathology reports	To create a system for extracting information from pathology reports with the purpose of storing the information in a research data warehouse	Pathology reports	The method is based on ML algorithm (i.e. sequence mapping)	International	Extraction of several fields from pathology reports with excellent accuracy
System13	Ni et al. (2014)	Increasing the efficiency of patient identification for clinical trials in the emergency department (ED)	To develop an automated eligibility screening (ES) approach for clinical trials in an urban tertiary care pediatric ED	Between January 1, 2010 and August 31, 2012, we gathered eligibility criteria for 13 diseases	Use the effectiveness of NLP, IE and ML techniques on real-world clinical data and trials	International	Researchers demonstrated that NLP-, IE- and ML-based automated ES could successfully select patients for clinical trials by using the text of trial criteria and the content of EHRs

System14	Bill et al. (2014)	Automated extraction of family history information from clinical notes	This paper describes the development and evaluation of a NLP module based on the unstructured information management application (UIMA) for automated extraction of family history information with functionality for identifying statements, observations, and prediction ("indicator phrases")	Sample of clinical notes	Use of UIMA (Unstructured Information Management Architecture) is a framework for an aging unstructured data	International	The family history NLP system achieved F-scores of 66.9, 92.4, 82.9, 57.3, 97.7 and 61.9
System15	McMurray et al. (2015)	Ontologically modeling of electronic health information exchange	Ontology was designed to measure and visualize regional interoperability	Data from are regional health system	Using Protégé 4, a knowledge-based framework and open-source web ontology language editor	International	Ontology was designed to measure and visualize regional interoperability

System16	Li et al. (2016)	A practical tool to implement hospital-based syndrome surveillance	The system discusses and examines the use of a symptom-clicking-module (SCM) as part of a hospital-based syndrome monitoring program	A total of 1,730,797 patient encounters were recorded by SCM	The clinicians used SCM to keep track of all of the patients who came in, and the data was automatically compiled and transmitted in daily batches. Using pre-defined criteria, the symptoms were grouped into seven targeted syndromes, and statistical techniques were used to detect temporal anomalies in the data series	International	Accuracy=92.1%

System17	Tripathi and Deshmukh (2017)	Building a database-driven reverse medical dictionary	The goal of the project was to create a fully complete reverse medical lexicon in order to improve the efficiency of health treatment consultations. Through an intelligent healthcare system, consumers can get rapid guidance on their health difficulties using a reverse medical vocabulary	User input is then the number of symptoms. Total inputs: 50	Use of three modules divided into three parts: preprocessing, filtering and ranking	Maharashtra	Accuracy=92%

System18	Jernite et al. (2013)	Predicting chief complaints at triage time in the emergency department	This study describes a method that helps achieve this objective by creating an extended ontology of chief complaints and automatically predicting a patient's top complaint based on their vitals and then users' description of their state upon arrival	A dataset of 97,000 triage notes	Use of linear support vector machine	International	Proposed a system for predicting a patient's main complaints based on a description of their current condition is good enough
System19	Usui et al. (2018)	Extraction and standardization of patient complaints from electronic medication histories for pharmacy covigilance	The goal of this study was to develop a system for collecting and standardizing patient complaints from computerized medication histories gathered data in Japanese community pharmacy in order to identify potential adverse drug event signals	A dataset of 5,000 patient complaints	Use of search rules on morphological analysis and speech	International	System performance was .66 regarding precision, .63 in recall and .65 for the F-measure

System20	Horng et al. (2019)	Modern ontology of emergency department presenting problem	Numerous attempts have been made to create a standardized "presenting problem" or "chief complaint" list to characterize the nature of an ED visit	A total of 180,424 patient visits were included in the study	Use of the hierarchical presenting problem ontology	International	Ontology successfully captured structured data for 95.9%.
System21	Barathi Ganesh et al. (2020)	Natural language understanding for medical texts	Natural language understanding is one of the essential tasks for building clinical text-based applications	Digital data in the form of clinical reports	Vector pace models are used, as well as sequential modeling jobs	National	Performance of 93.8% as the F1 score for i2b2 clinical corpus and achieves 97.29% as the F1 score for GENIA corpus
System22	Qing et al. (2019)	Neural network-based method for medical text classification	The approach creates sentence representations by combining two or more sentences. Dividing the document into segments and then combining them into a document representation.	Use of medical records	Use of neural networks	International	In this research, researcher suggests a novel hierarchical neural network method for medical text classification. Accuracy =Good

System23	Rousseau et al. (2019)	Data from emergency department	Comparing documentation on relevant clinical information in electronic health record (EHR). Providing note to computed tomography (CT) order requisition, prior to ordering of head CT for ED patients presenting with headache	Electronic health records	Performed between April 1, 2013 and September 30, 2014 at an adult quaternary academic hospital	International	Accuracy=90%
System24	Steinkamp et al. (2020)	Task definition, annotated dataset, and supervised natural language processing models for symptom extraction from unstructured clinical notes	ML and NLP have great potential to improve IE within electronic medical records for a wide variety of clinical search and summarization on tools	Use of 1,108 discharge summaries	For a clinically motivated symptom extraction ask, we present a task definition and detailed annotation requirements	International	The system is highly customizable to individual workflows and allows each user to choose which data should be structured and which should be unstructured

System25	Klyshinsky et al. (2020)	Formalization of medical records using ontology: patient complaints	Medical records contain a textual description of such important information as patients' complaints, diseases progress and therapy	Use of 100 medical records	To classify clinical statements into their assigned categories, a rule-based technique was applied	International	The algorithm corrects syntactical mistakes according to the hierarchical information from the ontology. The resulting algorithm was proved on 3,000 clinical records
System26	López-Úbeda et al. (2020)	An integrated approach to biomedical term identification systems	The authors present a unique architecture for developing biomedical term identification systems	Textual collections with clinical records	In order to construct the biomedical NER, we used certain NLP technologies. We begin by normalizing the content, which entails: removing punctuation, removing HTML elements, transforming the entire text to lowercase and coding it in UTF-8	International	BSB is an accurate system

System27	Yehia et al. (2019)	Ontology-based clinical IE from physician's free-text notes	An IE system that extracts structured data from handwritten clinical notes by physicians	The system is evaluated on real clinical notes	The OB-CIE system can help physicians to document visit notes without changing their workflow	International	F-measure of 94.90% and 97.80%
System28	Meystre et al. (2020)	Extracting information from textual documents in the electronic health record: a review of recent research	Examine recent published research on IE from textual documents in the electronic health record in this paper (EHR)	In this review, 174 papers were chosen and discussed	Literature review of the research published after 1995	International	Performance of IE systems with clinical text has improved since the last systematic review in 1995

System29	Lu et al. (2009)	Multilingual chief complaint classification for syndrome surveillance: An experiment with Chinese chief complaints	To ease data collection and analysis for automated syndrome surveillance, Chief Complaints must be grouped into established syndrome categories	Using statistical approaches, a set of 470 Chinese keywords was retrieved from around 1 million Chinese CC data	A novel Chinese CC classification system is proposed here, based on a Chinese–English translation module and an existing English CC classification on method	International	Accuracy=90%

System30	Wang et al. (2019)	Using natural language processing techniques to provide personalized educational materials for chronic disease patients in China: development and assessment of a knowledge-based health recommender system	The goal of this project was to create a health recommenders system in China that would deliver relevant teaching materials for chronic disease patients and assess its effectiveness	50 patients will be tested, and 100 educational documents will be distributed	Ontology and numerous NLP approaches were used to create a knowledge-based recommender system	International	A novel Chinese C classification system leveraging a Chinese–English translation module is better than others
System31	Lua et al. (2018)	Ontology-enhanced automatic chief complaint classification for syndromic surveillance	A new ontology-enhanced automatic CC classification approach is presented in this paper. In a medical ontology, using semantic relations	Real-world dataset	The UMLS-based weighted semantic similarity score (WSSS) grouping mechanism was used	International	Our ontology-enhanced strategy out performs the benchmark methods in terms of sensitivity, F-measure and F2 measure, according to his study

System32	Hier and Brint (2020)	A neuro-ontology for the neurological examination	Based on UMLS Met Thesaurus concepts, we investigated the feasibility of recording the neurological examination as machine-readable codes	A dataset of 2,386 test-cases was constructed based on 419 published neurological illnesses	Using 1,100 concepts from the UMLS Met thesaurus	International	The neurology examination ontology (NEO), which was created by combining different terminologies in UMLS
System33	Mall and Jaiswal (2018)	Survey of machine translation for Indian languages to English and its approaches	The purpose of this paper is to discuss the various methodologies used in translation systems for Indian languages to English languages	A total of 16 research papers on the conversion of Indian languages to English have been published	List the numerous MT approaches for converting Indian languages into other languages, as well as their advantages and disadvantages	National	Accuracy=80% For Indian language Hindi. Chunk performance is improved

System34	Dara et al. (2008)	Evaluation of preprocessing techniques for chief complaints	To see whether preparing a chief complaint before automatically categorizing them into syndrome groups improves classification accuracy	Using two preprocessors, chief complaints were preprocessed (CCP and EMT-P)	We preprocessed chief complaints using two preprocessors (CCP and EMT-P) and evaluated whether classification performance increased for a probabilistic classifier (CoCo)	International	CCP exhibited High accuracy=85% (chief complaint preprocessing)

System35	Mall and Jaiswal (2018)	Using chief complaints for syndrome surveillance: a review of chief complaint-based classifiers in North America (Mall and Jaiswal 2018)	This article examines 15 syndrome monitoring systems in North America, including those in cities, countries, states and the federal government	Reviewed 15 research papers	The studies on classifiers can be classified into two categories: statistical methods and keyword-based methods	International	All of the systems examined can be linked to respiratory and gastrointestinal disorders
System36	Dara et al. (2008)	Clinical information extraction applications: a literature review	A survey of the literature for clinical data extraction applications	There are 263 publications that have been thoroughly reviewed	A literature search was conducted using Ovid MEDLINE In-Process and other non-indexed citations, Ovid MEDLINE, OvidEMBASE, Scopus, Web of Science, and ACM Digital Library for publications published between January 2009 and September 2016	International	For title and abstract screening, a total of 1,917 publications were identified. 263 articles were chosen and discussed in this evaluation from among these publications

System37	Hansoti et al. (2021)	Calibrating a chief complaint list for lower source settings: a methodological case study	This research was done as part of a wider prospective observational study on human immune deficiency virus testing in South African emergency departments	Paper case report forms were used to collect data on 3,357 patients	The frequency of concordance between the coded chief complaint word and the selected symptom(s) from the pilot symptom list was determined by two members of the study team	International	A systematic process for calibrating a chief complaint list or the local context was described in this study
System38	Musa et al. (2014)	Ontology knowledge map for enhancing healthcare services: a case of emergency unit of specialist hospital	It offers an ontology knowledge map-based strategy for locating superfluous us transactions that need to be modified in order to improve healthcare administration	Use of electronic health records	We chose the ontology as the study's base because it is thought to be capable of providing a better understanding of an organization dynamics, allowing for a good alignment between enterprise design and operation, and allowing for a systematic reengineer plan	National	One of the ways commended is to automate the emergency departments by introducing EHR systems, which will make it easier for the actors in the unit to rapidly and accurately obtain all of the information they need about a patient

System39	Elmessiry et al. (2017)	Medical diagnosis by complaints of patients and ML	The objective is to identify a link between the patient's complaints and probable diseases	Dataset of 10,000 authorial medical website	The key to detecting correlations between patients' complaints and probable diseases is to use ML models, as describe d in this research	International	Accuracy=75% Precision=81% Recall=81%
System40	Elmessiry et al. (2017)	Leveraging sentiment analysis for classifying patient complaints	The goal of this study is to automate the classification of patient complaints in order to enhance triage and response times	Use of electronic health records	Using increased linguistic inquiry and a word count lexicon, map each complaint to a vector	International	Accuracy=84%

Table 9.3. *Summary of approaches and contribution*

9.4. Results and discussion

19 of the 40 potential research projects were methodology-based, five were technique-based, three were framework-based, five were process-based and eight were assessments of existing projects. The methods taken into account are ontology-based, as shown in Table 9.3, and they involve the usage of the Protégé–owl editor tool, Protégé 4, OWL 2, OWL and SNOMED CT. The main contributions include, but are not limited to: modeling of protégé-based knowledge representation for linking concepts and data for diabetes diseases; mobile-based healthcare ontology; classification of diseases based on phenotypes; advancement in service provision and accessibility to trustworthy health data. Table 9.4 displays the findings of the review. A graphical representation is shown in Figure 9.3. This provides an overview of the number of studies per initiative that were located and shows the data about the functions intended to enhance healthcare operational procedures. These characteristics can serve as the foundation for approaches, frameworks, workflows, methodologies and reviews.

System number	System name	Types of initiative	Type of method/tech./process/frame/ review
System1	Syndrome Biosurveillance system (Chapman et al. 2005)	Method	Experimental
System2	SNOMED clinical system (Patrick et al. 2007)	Method	Experimental
System3	SNOMED clinical information management (Patrick et al. 2007)	Method	Experimental

System4	Evaluation of preprocessing techniques for chief complaint classification (Dara et al. 2008)	Process	Process mapping: use of two preprocessors (CCP and EMT-P)
System5	Automatic segmentation of clinical texts (Apostolova et al. 2009)	Method	Experiment setup: rule-based algorithm
System6	A medication information extraction system for clinical narratives (Xu et al. 2010)	Method	Mixed method
System7	Classification of free-text clinical narratives (Kaurova et al. 2011)	Review	Systematic review
System8	Natural language processing systems for capturing and standardizing unstructured clinical information: A systematic review (Kreimeyer et al. 2017)	Review	Systematic review
System9	Developing ontology for data quality in chronic disease (Rahimi et al. 2012)	Technique	Developed an ontological toolkit to support research and quality improvement studies

System10	A review of chief complaint-based classifiers in North America (Conway et al. 2013)	Review	Literature review
System11	A priority for global emergency care research in low-income countries (Mowafi et al. 2019)	Review	Systematic review
System12	The pathology extraction pipeline for information extraction from pathology reports (Ashish et al. 2014)	Process	Sequence mapping
System13	Increasing the efficiency of patient identification for clinical trials in the emergency department (Ni et al. 2014)	Technique	Use of leveraging natural language processing, information extraction and machine learning technologies
System14	Automated extraction of family history information from clinical notes (Bill et al. 2014)	Framework	Unstructured information management architecture
System15	Ontological modeling of electronic health information exchange (McMurray et al. 2015)	Framework	Conceptual framework

System16	A practical tool to implement hospital based syndrome surveillance (Li et al. 2016)	Process	Sequential mapping
System17	Building a database-driven reverse medical dictionary (Tripathi and Deshmukh 2017)	Method	Experimental
System18	Predicting chief complaints at triage time in the emergency department (Jernite et al. 2013)	Method	Experimental
System19	Extraction and standardization of patient complaints from electronic medication histories for pharmacy covigilance (Usui et al. 2018)	Method	Experimental
System20	Modern ontology of emergency department presenting problems (Horng et al. 2019)	Method	Classification
System21	Natural language understand for medical texts (Barathi Ganesh et al. 2020)	Framework	Linear

System22	Neural network-based method for medical text classification (Qing et al. 2019)	Method	Experimental
System23	Automated retrieval of data from emergency department (Rousseau et al. 2019)	Method	Observational
System24	Task definition, annotated dataset, and supervised natural language processing models for symptom extraction from unstructured clinical notes (Steinkamp et al. 2020)	Techniques	Develop model for symptom extraction from unstructured clinical notes
System25	Formalization of medical records using ontology: Patient complaints (Klyshinsky et al. 2020)	Method	Experimental
System26	An integrated approach to biomedical term identification systems (López-Úbeda et al. 2020)	Framework	Modular-based
System27	Ontology-based clinical information extraction from physician's free-text notes (Yehia et al. 2019)	Process	Rule-based

System28	Extracting information from textual documents in the electronic health record: A review of recent research (Meystre et al. 2020)	Review	Systematic review
System29	Multilingual chief complaint classification for syndromic surveillance: An experiment with Chinese chief complaints (Lu et al. 2009)	Method	Experimental
System30	Using natural language processing techniques to provide personalized educational materials for chronic disease patients in China: Development and assessment of a knowledge-based health recommender system (Wang et al. 2019)	Technique	Rule-based approach
System31	Ontology-enhanced automatic chief complaint classification for syndromic surveillance (Lua et al. 2018)	Method	This paper uses two popular CC classification methods using a real-world dataset
System32	A neuro-ontology for the neurological examination (Hier and Brint 2020)	Method	Use of ontology

System33	Survey of machine translation for Indian languages to English and its approaches (Mall and Jaiswal 2018)	Review	Review on 16 research papers
System34	Evaluation of preprocessing techniques for chief complaints (Dara et al. 2008)	Process	We preprocessed chief complaints using two preprocessors (CCP and EMT-P)
System35	Using chief complaints for syndromic surveillance: A review of chief complaint-based classifiers in North America (Mall and Jaiswal 2018)	Review	Review on 15 research papers
System36	Clinical information extraction applications: A literature review (Dara et al. 2008)	Review	Review 263 articles selected for review
System37	Calibrating a chief complaint list for lower source settings: A methodological case study (Hansoti et al. 2021)	Method	Paper presents methodological strategy that can be exported to other settings to refine a local chief complaint list
System38	Ontology knowledge map for enhancing healthcare services: A case of emergency unit of specialist hospital (Musa et al. 2014)	Method	Method-based ontology

System39	Medical diagnosis by complaints of patients and machine learning (Elmessiry et al. 2017)	Technique	Machine learning
System40	Leveraging sentiment analysis for classifying patient complaints	Method	Vector-based

Table 9.4. *Summary of quantity of studies per initiative*

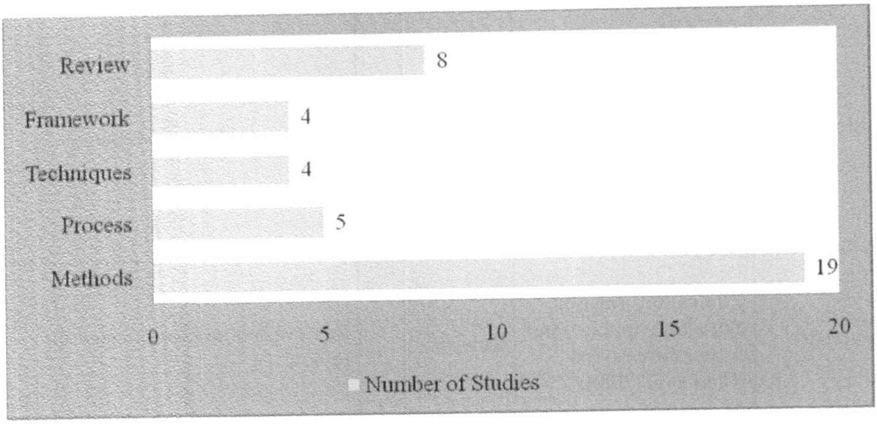

Figure 9.3. *Summary of quantity of studies per initiative discovered. For a color version of this figure, see www.iste.co.uk/pradhan/cognitivecomputing.zip*

9.5. Conclusion

The available literature on the use of NLP in healthcare was compiled in this review. This helps to provide researchers in the sector with complete information about currently used approaches, improvements to the caliber of healthcare services, and limitations. It included information on the goals of particular researchers as well as their contributions to enhancing healthcare through the use of NLP, and the restrictions placed on their research. It was also shown that several researchers in this field used a range of strategies to enhance healthcare through NLP. Some approaches used particular methodologies, techniques, procedures and frameworks, while others were modifications of those that previously existed. This healthcare

NLP review identified the requirement for ontology-based models to enhance the delivery of healthcare services for both patients and healthcare providers. Researchers in the field of NLP in healthcare can use this study's findings to pinpoint any gaps or problem areas. As a result, the research field will contribute even more.

9.6. References

Apostolova, E., Channin, D., Fushman, D.D., Lytinen, S.L., Stan Raicu, D. (2009). Automatic segmentation of clinical texts. *Annu. Int. Conf. IEEE Eng. Med. Biol. Soc.*, 5905–8. doi: 10.1109/IEMBS.2009.5334831.

Ashish, N., Dahm, L.M., Boicey, C.M. (2014). Pathology extraction pipeline: The pathology extraction pipeline for information extraction from pathology reports. *Health Informatics Journal*, 20(4), 288–305. doi: 10.1177/1460458213494032.

Barathi Ganesh, H.B., Reshma, U., Soman, K.P., Anand Kumar, M. (2020). Med NLU: Natural language understander for medical texts. In *Deep Learning Techniques for Biomedical and Health Informatics*, Dash, S., Acharya, B., Mittal, M., Abraham, A., Kelemen, A. (eds). Springer, Cham. doi: 10.1007/978-3-030-33966-1_1.

Bill, R., Pakhomov, S., Chen, E.S., Winden, T.J., Carter, E.W., Melton, G.B. (2014). Automated extraction of family history information from clinical notes. *AMIA Annu. Symp. Proc.*, 1709–1717.

Chapman, W.W., Christensen, L.M., Wagner, M.M., Haug, P.J., Ivanov, O., Dowling, J.N., Olszewski, R.T. (2005). Classifying free-text triage chief complaints into syndrome categories with natural language processing. *Artif. Intell. Med.*, 33(1), 31–40.

Conway, M., Dowling, J.N., Chapman, W.W. (2013). Using chief complaints for syndrome surveillance: Are view of chief complaint based classifiers in North America. *J. Biomed. Inform.*, 46(4), 734–743.

Cyrus, J.W. (2014). A review of recent research on internet access, use, and on line health information seeking. *Journal of Hospital Librarianship*, 14(2), 149–157.

Dahm, M.R. (2012). Tales of time, terms, and patient information-seeking behavior—an exploratory qualitative study. *Health Communication*, 27(7), 682–689.

Dara, J., Dowling, J.N., Travers, D., Cooper, G.F., Chapman, W.W. (2008). Evaluation of preprocessing techniques for chief complaint classification. *Journal of Biomedical Informatics*, 41, 613–623.

Elmessiry, A., Zhang, Z., Cooper, W.O., Catron, T.F., Karrass, J., Singh, M.P. (2017). Leveraging sentiment analysis for classifying patient complaints. *Proceedings of the 8th ACM International Conference on Bioinformatics, Computational Biology, and Health Informatics*, 44–51.

Esteva, A., Robicquet, A., Ramsundar, B., Kuleshov, V., De Pristo, M., Chou, K., Dean, J. (2019). A guide to deeplearning in healthcare. *Nature Medicine*, 25(1), 24–29.

Gupta, A., Lai, A., Mozersky, J., Ma, X., Walsh, H., DuBois, J.M. (2021). Enabling qualitative research data sharing using a natural language processing pipeline for deidentification: Moving beyond HIPAA Safe Harbor identifiers. *JAMIA Open*, 4(3). doi: 10.1093/jamiaopen/ooab069.

Hansoti, B., Hahn, E., Rao, A., Harris, J., Jenson, A., Markadakis, N., Moonat, S., Osula, V., Pousson, A. (2021). Calibrating a chief complaint list for low resource settings: A methodological case study. *Int. J Emerg. Med.*, 14(1), 32.

Hier, D.B. and Brint, S.U. (2020). A neuro-ontology for the neurological examination. *BMC Medical Informatics and Decision Making*, 20, 47.

Horng, S., Greenbaum, N.R., Nathanson, L.A., McClay, J.C., Goss, F.R., Nielson, J.A. (2019). Consensus development of a modern ontology of emergency department presenting problems. *Appl. Clin. Inform.*, 10(3), 409–420.

Jernite, Y., Halpern, Y., Horng, S., Sontag, D. (2013). Predicting chief complaints at triage time in the emergency department. *NIPS 2013 Workshop on Machine Learning for Clinical Data Analysis and Healthcare*.

Kaurova, O., Alexandrov, M., Blanco, X. (2011). Classification of free text clinical narratives (short review). *Business and Engineering Applications of Intelligent and Information Systems*, 124.

Keifenheim, K.E., Teufel, M., Ip, J., Speiser, N., Leehr, E.J., Zipfel, S., Herrmann-Werner, A. (2015). Teaching history taking to medical students: A systematic review. *BMC Medical Education*, 15(1), 159.

Kitchenham, B. (2004). Procedures for performing systematic reviews. Technical Report, Keele University, 33.

Klyshinsky, E.S., Gribova, V.V., Shakhgeldyan, C., Shalfeeva, E.A., Okun, D., Geltser, B.I., Gorbach, T.A., Karpik, O.D. (2020). Formalization of medical records using an ontology: Patient complaints. In *Analysis of Images, Social Networks and Texts*, van der Aalst, W.M.P., Batagelj, V., Ignatov, D.I. et al. (eds). Springer, Cham, 143–153.

Kreimeyer, K., Foster, M., Pandey, A., Arya, N., Halford, G., Jones, S.F., Forshee, R., Walderhaug, M., Botsis, T. (2017). Natural language processing systems for capturing and standardizing unstructured clinical information: A systematic review. *Journal of Biomedical Informatics*, 73, 14–29.

Li, G., Song, H., Liang, H.-N., Qu, Y., Liu, L., Bai, X. (2019). Medical diagnosis by complaints of patients and machine learning. *2019 12th International Congress on Image and Signal Processing, BioMedical Engineering and Informatics (CISP-BMEI)*, Suzhou, 1–5. doi: 10.1109/CISP-BMEI48845.2019.8965949.

López-Úbeda, P., Díaz-Galiano, M.C., Montejo-Ráez, A., Martín-Valdivia, M.T. (2020). An integrated approach to biomedical term identification systems. *Appl. Sci.*, 10(5), 1726.

Lu, H.-M., Chen, H., Zeng, D., King, C.-C., Shih, F.-Y., Wu, T.-S., Hsiao, J.-Y. (2009). Multilingual chief complaint classification for syndrome surveillance: An experiment with Chinese chief complaints. *Int. J Med. Inform.*, 78(5), 308–320.

Lua, H.-M., Zengab, D., Trujilloc, L., Komatsuc, K., Chena, H. (2008). Ontology-enhanced automatic chief complaint classification or syndromic surveillance. *J. Biomed. Inform.*, 41(2), 340–356.

Mall, S. and Jaiswal, U.C. (2018). Survey: Machine translation for Indian language. *International Journal of Applied Engineering Research*, 13(1), 202-209.

McMurray, J., Zhu, L., McKillop, I., Chen, H. (2015). Ontological modeling of electronic health information exchange. *Journal of Biomedical Informatics*, 56, 169–178.

Meuter, R.F., Gallois, C., Segalowitz, N.S., Ryder, A.G., Hocking, J. (2015). Overcoming language barriers in healthcare: A protocol for investigating a few and effective communication when patients or clinicians use a second language. *BMC Health Services Research*, 15(1), 371.

Meystre, S.M., Savova, G., Kipper-Schuler, K.C., Hurdle, J.F. (2020). Extracting information from textual documents in the electronic health record: A review of recent research. *Yearb. Med. Inform.*, 128–144.

Mowafi, H., Workis, D.D., Bisanzo, M., Hansoti, B., Seidenberg, P., Obermeyer, Z., Hauswald, M., Reynolds, T.A. (2019). Making recording and analysis of chief complaint a priority for global emergency care research in low-income countries. *Acad. Emerg. Med.*, 20(12), 1241–1245.

Musa, M., Othman, M., Al-Rahimi, W.M. (2014). Ontology knowledge map for enhancing health care services: A case of emergency unit of specialist hospital. *Journal of Theoretical and Applied Information Technology*, 70, 196–209.

Ni, Y., Kennebeck, S., Dexheimer, J.W., McAneney, C.M., Tang, H., Lingren, T., Li, Q., Zhai, H., Solti, I. (2014). Automated clinical trial eligibility prescreening: Increasing the efficiency of patient identification for clinical trials in the emergency department. *J. Am. Med. Inform. Assoc.*, 22(1), 166–78.

Patrick, J., Wang, Y., Budd, P. (2007). An automated system for conversion of clinical notes into SNOMED clinical terminology. *Proceedings of the fifth Australasian symposium on ACSW frontiers*, Ballarat, 68, 219–226.

Qing, L., Linhong, W., Xuehai, D. (2019). A novel neural network-based method for medical text classification. *Future Internet*, 11, 12.

Rahimi, A., Liaw, S.-T., Taggart, J., Ray, P., Yu, H. (2012). Developing ontology for data quality in chronic disease management. *International Journal of E-Health and Medical Communications*, 5(3), 58–77. doi: 10.4018/ijehmc.2014070105.

Rousseau, J.F., Ip, I.K., Raja, A.S., Valtchinov, V.I., Cochon, L., Schuur, J.D., Khorasani, R. (2019). Can automated retrieval of data from emergency department physician notes enhance the imaging order entry process? *Appl. Clin. Inform.*, 10(2), 189–198.

Silverman, J., Kurtz, S., Draper, J. (2016). *Skills for Communicating with Patients*. CRC Press, Boca Raton.

Steinkamp, J.M., Bala, W., Sharma, A., Kantrowitz, J.J. (2020). Task definition, annotated dataset, and supervised natural language processing models for symptom extraction from unstructured clinical notes. *J. Biomed. Inform.*, 102, 103354. doi: 10.1016/j.jbi.2019.103354.

Tripathi, P. and Deshmukh, M. (2017). Building a scalable database driven reverse medical dictionary using NLP techniques. *Advances in Computational Sciences and Technology*, 10(5), 1221–1231.

Usui, M., Aramaki, E., Iwao, T., Wakamiya, S., Sakamoto, T., Mochizuki, M. (2018). Extraction and standardization of patient complaints from electronic medication histories for pharma covigilance: Natural language processing analysis in Japanese. *JMIR. Med. Inform.*, 6(3), e11021.

Van Rosse, F., de Bruijne, M., Suurmond, J., Essink-Bot, M.L., Wagner, C. (2016). Language barriers and patient safety risks in hospital care. A mixed methods study. *International Journal of Nursing Studies*, 54, 45–53.

Wagholikar, A.S., Lawley, M.J., Hansen. P., Chu, K. (2011). Identifying symptom groups from emergency department presenting complaint free text using SNOMED CT. *AMIA Annual Symposium Proceedings*, 1446.

Wang, Z., Huang, H., Cui, L., Chen, J., An, J., Duan, H., Ge, H., Deng, N. (2019). Using natural language processing techniques to provide personalized educational materials for chronic disease patients in china: development and assessment of a knowledge-based health recommender system. *JMIR. Med. Inform.*, 8(4), e17642. doi: 10.2196/17642.

Xu, H., Stenner, S.P., Doan, S., Johnson, K.B., Waitman, L.R., Denny, J.C. (2010). MedEx: A medication information extraction system for clinical narratives. *J. Am. Med. Inform. Assoc.*, 17(1), 19–24.

Ye, C., Li, Z., Fu, Y., Lan, Y., Zhu, W., Zhou, D., Zhang, H., Lai, H.Z.S., Buckeridge, D.L., Sun, Q. et al. (2016). SCM: A practical tool to implement hospital based syndrome surveillance. *BMC Res Notes* 9, 315. doi: 10.1186/s13104-016-2098-z.

Yehia, E., Boshnak, H., Abdel, S., Amany, G., Doaa, A., Elzanfaly, S. (2019). Ontology-based clinical information extraction from physician's free-text notes. *Journal of Biomedical Informatics*, 98, 103276.

Young, T., Hazarika, D., Poria, S., Cambria, E. (2018). Recent trends in deep learning based natural language processing. *IEEE Computational Intelligence Magazine*, 13(3), 55–75.

10

Artificial Intelligence and Large Language Models in Mental Healthcare: A Systematic Review

Artificial intelligence (AI) in the mental health sector is proving to be a game changer in providing more effective and individualized treatment programs. Recent studies in AI-based mental healthcare have paid attention to the benefits and ethical considerations of this experience. This chapter presents a comprehensive review of the literature on the ethical application of AI in mental healthcare. The results indicate that multiple studies observed a positive effect of AI-based mental healthcare through machine learning (ML), chatbots and AI-based MH-apps. However, these benefits are gradually diminishing due to the need for more ethical considerations. It was also found that research demonstrating the combination of in-person mental healthcare and AI-based mental healthcare is limited.

10.1. Introduction

Mental health is not only the absence of mental illness or disorder, but also a positive state of being that enables individuals to thrive and achieve their goals (Keyes 2002). It consists of many factors, such as emotional regulation, social connections, resilience and a sense of purpose in life.

For a long time, traditional mental health encompassing face-to-face therapy has been delivered in various ways, such as psychological therapies, like cognitive, behavioral and psychotherapy. Moreover, somatic therapies such as medicines and

Chapter written by Mansi CHITGOPEKAR, Abdul Raffie NAIK and Mahimna VYAS.

electroconvulsive therapy have also played an integral part in aiding individuals with mental health issues.

Moreover, how mental health treatment can be offered today has shown significant development, even though conventional methods have a wealth of empirical support and excellent validity and reliability (Kazdin and Blase 2011). One of the most remarkable methods is artificial intelligence (AI). The application of AI within the mental health sector could be of great assistance as it is known for effective and personalized treatment plans. AI has access to massive dataset collections that can help researchers understand what makes some people more vulnerable to mental illness, improve diagnostic precision and further determine who benefits from specific therapies.

Additionally, by providing individualized and data-driven therapeutic approaches, AI can fundamentally change psychological treatment modalities (Pereira et al. 2021). AI can be used to create virtual therapists that can offer assistance and direction to people struggling with mental health concerns (Lee et al. 2021). AI is used in psychology to develop chatbots that can offer automated support and direction to people needing mental health services (Liu et al. 2022). Based on the user's input, these chatbots can be trained to use natural language processing to offer sympathetic answers and individualized guidance.

Artificial intelligence (AI) has immense potential to enhance access and reduce consumer costs, but several challenges exist. In recent years, AI has been increasingly used in psychology to support patients, similar to in-person therapy. With the increase in Covid-19 and its associated stressors, multiple organizations have turned to AI to increase the availability and accessibility of mental health services (Liu et al. 2022).

However, AI-based mental health support has some drawbacks associated with it. Data security and privacy are among the most prominent disadvantages (Mann et al. 2021). For many AI services, businesses acquire, manage and use data. This data is accessible to private organizations, medical facilities and government agencies. The possibility of data leaking to other parties or hackers always exists (Gerke et al. 2020). In addition, using AI to make decisions regarding diagnosis and treatment without enough human oversight and input raises issues (Mörch et al. 2020). To ensure that the technology is used in a responsible and secure manner, ethical norms and standards should be applied to guide the usage of AI in psychology.

Furthermore, the possibility of bias in AI algorithms, which could result in bias against specific groups, is thus one of the main ethical concerns (Fiske et al. 2019). For example, an AI algorithm may offer biased treatment suggestions if trained on data not representative of the community. Another ethical issue is the prospect of AI being used in ways that violate patients' rights to confidentiality and privacy (Grainger and Sikka 2020). The privacy and confidentiality of the patients must be protected, and the data must only be used for the intended reasons when AI systems that analyze sensitive patient data are created.

Thus, the global mental health system is already overworked due to increased instances and a shortage of healthcare workers to handle the cases. The demand and supply are significantly out of balance. People are increasingly turning to digital solutions to address mental health difficulties as knowledge of the problem grows. The use of AI in the field of mental health is just beginning. AI is anticipated to significantly contribute to managing mental health as technology develops and public awareness rises. However, AI in treatment modalities in the mental health sector has a major ethical implication that must be addressed to ensure that technology is used responsibly and safely.

10.1.1. *Objectives*

– To understand the effect of AI-based assessment, diagnosis or intervention on individuals with mental health disorders.

– To understand whether AI gives the same support and connectivity as in-person therapy.

– To compare the credibility of AI-based mental health support to in-person mental healthcare.

– To investigate the ethical issues raised in AI-based mental healthcare.

10.1.2. *Methods*

For this systematic review, a search was conducted through multiple electronic literature databases such as PubMed, APA PsychInfo, Science Direct, EMBASE Psych, Google Scholar, Web of Science and science gate. These databases were searched using a predetermined set of keywords. These keywords were modified to reflect the finding and thus ensure relevance to the research. Under these databases, research papers and articles published in English on AI and mental health were searched. Under mental health as the umbrella term, the authors also included multiple subtopics, such as various disorders and their relationship with AI (e.g. AI and depression, AI and bipolar disorder), helping the authors gain research papers that were more specific and detailed. The data used were extracted from published articles only. The process of selecting a study primarily depended on the abstract. If the abstract depicted research on a relationship between mental health or any disorder and AI, then it was selected, and the entire research paper was analyzed.

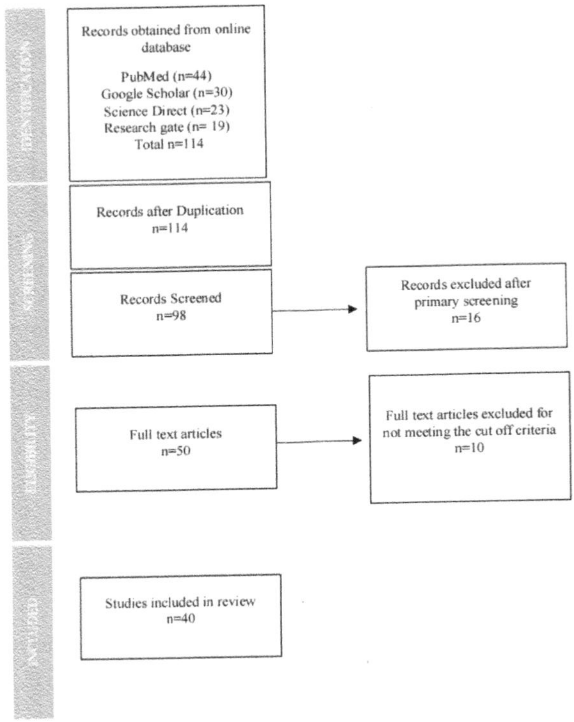

Figure 10.1. *Prisma flowchart. For a color version of this figure, see www.iste.co.uk/pradhan/cognitivecomputing.zip*

10.1.3. *Inclusion criteria*

– Studies with various forms of AI (i.e. chatbots, ML, MH-apps, etc.) were included to understand the effectiveness and concerns of various forms of AI.

– Studies conducted in different countries to gain a diverse range of data from various populations, further leading to a high generalization of the results of this chapter.

– Studies focusing on various mental health disorders such as anxiety, depression, bipolar disorder, developmental disorders, schizophrenia and other related disorders.

– Studies that are published in the English Language.

10.1.4. *Exclusion criteria*

– Studies that do not use various forms of AI for diagnosis, treatment or assessment.

– Studies that are not published in English.

10.1.5. *Discussion*

This chapter covers the current research on AI-based mental health intervention worldwide over the past 10 years, as well as what is known about the characteristics of AI in the field of mental healthcare. It increases our understanding of advancements and developments in the mental health field while highlighting the scope and gravity of the ethical issues and constraints that AI introduces.

This chapter highlights the diversity of AI-based mental healthcare used in various studies and research papers, along with their findings, advantages and limitations.

10.2. AI as an advantage for users

Artificial intelligence is widely recognized for development in the mental health field. Along with professional support, AI has been recently recognized for the various advantages it gives to the users. The AI-care system has been assessed based on its feasibility and clinical usefulness, significantly improving clinical outcomes and reducing healthcare costs (Thermolia et al. 2015). Moreover, AI-assisted online social therapy that was based on an AI called rebound which was designed to deliver cognitive behavioral therapy (CBT) in a mental health app was found to be used for a randomized control trial, wherein the users provided feedback post as 12 week-program, mentioning the app to be feasible and acceptable to the participants. Most of the users reported high satisfaction with the program. Additionally, individuals reported an improvement in their mental health, a reduction in symptoms of anxiety and depression, and an advancement in social functioning (D'Alfonso et al. 2017). AI can be underlined to showcase its potential as an accessible therapeutic agent, being an effective and scalable intervention in mental healthcare (Fulmer et al. 2018).

Mental healthcare is readily available on an individual's phone. Nowadays, almost every individual has access to an electronic device. Thus, AI-based mental health mobile apps are readily available, making them widely accessible, in addition to being able to provide personalized interventions and monitor user symptoms in real time (Gamble 2020). Personalizing mental health therapies with AI can improve involvement and enhance outcomes for those with depression and anxiety. However, it should be mentioned that further study is required to improve AI algorithms and make sure they are ethically and efficiently used (Jacobson and Nemesure 2021).

AI care has been provided to users in multiple forms (i.e. chatbots, MH-apps, ML, etc.) that have been well received and perceived by users and are further considered to be helpful. Multiple users reported a reduction in symptoms of anxiety and depression, thus giving an insight into acceptability and effectiveness (Mehta et al. 2021). In a randomized control trial on AI-based emotional regulation and psychological intervention in middle school individuals, the students reported improved emotional regulation and decreased negative emotions (Wang et al. 2022).

Given the rising frequency of mental health concerns and the shortage of mental health practitioners, AI-based interventions can help close the gap and offer support to those who cannot have access to conventional mental healthcare.

10.3. Ethical implications of AI

Artificial intelligence in mental healthcare involves concerns regarding privacy, autonomy and fairness that are morally reprehensible. Some ethical issues arise from the acquisition and use of delicate personal data, such as that pertaining to our physical and mental well-being, which necessitates careful consideration of privacy protections and data security measures. Although embodied AI can potentially enhance mental health services, it raises several ethical issues that must be resolved. It further underlines the need for standards and laws to ensure that the development and implementation of embodied AI technologies in mental healthcare conform to ethical values and protect patient safety and well-being (Fiskeet et al. 2019).

The Canada Protocol is an ethical guideline for using AI in mental health and suicide prevention. It raises ethical questions about data protection, privacy, informed permission and potential biases in AI algorithms. It establishes a framework for the ethical development, use and assessment of AI-based therapies for mental health and suicide prevention (Mörch et al. 2020).

Although embodied AI has the potential to enhance mental health services, it also raises a number of ethical issues that must be resolved, further underlining the need for standards and laws to ensure that the development and implementation of embodied AI technologies in mental healthcare conform to ethical values and protect patient safety and well-being (Owusu et al. 2021). The emerging area of digital psychiatry and its potential impact on mental health treatment demonstrates the challenges and limitations of these approaches, including concerns about data privacy, regulation and the need for further study and evaluation of their effectiveness (Torous et al. 2021). The necessity for ethical concerns, the possibility of bias in AI algorithms and the significance of preserving a human connection in treatment are some of the potential risks and limitations of using AI in mental healthcare (Zhang et al. 2021).

Considering the closeness and daily engagement it has with patients or users regularly, ethical concern thus plays a significant role in the development of AI in the field of psychology.

10.4. AI chatbot and its functions in diagnosing and intervention

Without the help of a real therapist, chatbots in the field of mental health offer a means for people to get assistance and direction. They can be accessed at any time, provide personalized responses and offer a sense of anonymity, which can appeal to people who feel embarrassed or stigmatized about getting help from an in-person therapist. In a randomized controlled experiment with 70 participants, the effectiveness of an AI chatbot in lowering symptoms of anxiety and depression was investigated. Compared to the control group, the experimental group's depression and anxiety symptoms significantly decreased (Fulmer et al. 2018).

Digital psychiatry's modern technological capabilities are revolutionizing mental healthcare in intriguing new ways and potentially advancing future mental health research and care (Torous et al. 2021). Adults with depressive and anxiety symptoms can benefit from chatbot-delivered psychotherapy; however, the effectiveness varies between chatbot programs. Chatbots have been proven to moderately impact symptom reduction in depression and anxiety disorders (Lim et al. 2021). Moreover, an AI-based chatbot pilot study that was randomized and controlled was created to assist university students in managing their anxiety and depression. There were signs of potential efficacy, and the chatbot was deemed to be a suitable intervention (Klos et al. 2021).

The provision of mental healthcare in a range of AI-powered interventions, including chatbots, smartphone apps and virtual reality, has the potential to significantly improve the results for a variety of mental health issues such as depression and anxiety (Liu et al. 2022). The chatbot offered users information on self-help techniques for depression and encouraging and understanding answers, according to an evaluation of its messages and their efficacy in delivering evidence-based therapies for depression, highlighting the widespread use of chatbots in the mental health sector (Martinengo et al. 2022).

10.5. Machine learning as a base of AI for mental healthcare

Machine learning has become a promising tool in mental health. It is used for individualized treatment for people with mental health problems.

Machine learning in the field of mental healthcare has worked in various domains and explored depression, anxiety and schizophrenia. The various types of data used in ML models are behavioral, physiological and text data. ML techniques have been applied in the mental health field for predicting responses, detecting suicide risks and identifying trajectories. Despite it needing rigorous evaluation, ML showcases the potential to transform mental healthcare (Thieme et al. 2020). Prediction of anxiety and depression in people with immune-mediated inflammatory illnesses using ML algorithms has been studied for an extended period. According to the findings, these models could predict depression and anxiety in this population with moderate to high accuracy (Tennenhouse et al. 2020). However, ML-based models on pretreatment symptoms and electroencephalographic characteristics tend to have a moderate accuracy in predicting the outcome of antidepressant treatment in adults with depression (Rajpurkar et al. 2020).

ML methods have further shown that these models can predict the treatment outcomes of using antidepressant medications on patients with a moderate level of accuracy and additionally can improve clinical decision-making and individualized form of treatment (Nunez et al. 2021). ML and emotional AI (EAI) can improve the accuracy and reliability of depression detection and suggest that using these technologies can help overcome some of the limitations of traditional screening methods (Joshi and Kanoongo 2022). AI and ML are accelerated with use in mental health apps, although more research is essential to assess their effectiveness and address ethical concerns about their increasing use (Milne-Ives et al. 2022). With an overall accuracy of 76.2%, ML models can predict the treatment response in major depressive disorder. Comparing EEG measurements to clinical or demographic factors, it was discovered that the former was a superior indicator of therapy response (Watts et al. 2022).

However, the ethical issues surrounding the application of ML to mental health must be acknowledged, and the significance of informed consent, privacy protection and openness towards users must be emphasized.

10.6. Forms of AI as a mental healthcare support mechanism

AI-based mental healthcare is offered in many ways, including chatbots and ML. However, numerous more kinds have significantly aided the mental health sector. AI care is a clinical decision support system for the management of bipolar disorder. It applies AI algorithms to offer patients with bipolar disorder individualized treatment recommendations, moreover indicating that the approach has the potential to save healthcare costs while improving patient outcomes (Thermolia et al. 2015). Eheadspace is an AI-aided online social therapy program that uses natural language processing (NLP) to offer users individualized support and feedback during online social therapy sessions with a certified clinician. The results suggest AI-assisted online social therapy programs as a potentially promising means of providing young people access to high-quality mental healthcare (D'Alfonso et al. 2017). To distinguish between bipolar and unipolar depression, functional and structural MRI scans were used. Establishing that, in contrast to individuals with unipolar depression, patients with bipolar depression displayed significant variations in regional gray matter volumes and functional connectivity (Han et al. 2019).

Social media and AI usage have increased significantly in the mental health sector. Novel concepts for digital autonomy in the healthcare field have emerged as an outcome. It sheds light on the possible advantages and difficulties of using social media and AI in the context of depression and how they relate to digital autonomy (Laacke et al. 2021). Additionally, using the Deep Learning-aided Integrated Prediction Model (DLIPM), mental illness in children can be predicted and identified early on. With a high sensitivity rate of 97.9%, specificity rate of 96.7%, recall ratio of 95.6%, precision ratio of 90.1% and a lower error rate of 9.2%, the model outperforms other existing techniques, hence providing information about developing various types of AI support for mental healthcare (Zhang et al. 2021).

Based on an extensive analysis of the data from a range of AI technologies, such as computer vision, natural language processing and ML, it was discovered that AI-driven technologies had shown promising outcomes in the diagnosis of several mental disorders, including schizophrenia, depression and anxiety (Alaa Abd-Alrazaq et al. 2022). The use of emotion AI in the commercial sector and its implications in the mental health field provide into the present and prospective future of emotion AI. The monitoring and interpreting users' emotional states are becoming more common in consumer technology products, such as wearable technologies, chatbots and virtual assistants, showing the broad application of AI based on mental health (Monteith et al. 2022).

Consequently, this gives an insight into the many different ways that AI is used in the field of mental health. However, it should be noted that a significant amount of research is needed to determine the reliability, validity and ethical consideration of these support mechanisms.

10.7. AI as a support for mental health professional

There is growing interest in the application of AI in the field of mental health to help professionals provide mental healthcare. According to a study, digital phenotyping using smartphone data can accurately predict relapses in schizophrenia patients, emphasizing the potential of digital tools to enhance clinical treatment of mental health issues (Barnett et al. 2018). Consequently, it serves as a crucial aid agent for mental health professionals. ML techniques have demonstrated effectiveness in enhancing the precision of depression diagnosis and subtyping and predicting treatment effects. Additional research is required to determine the clinical significance (Gao et al. 2018). The diagnosis and management of mental health diseases could be improved by ML. However, the need for transparency, accountability, informed consent and other ethical and practical issues related to the application of ML in mental health must be considered (Shatte et al. 2019).

Moreover, AI and social media platforms in the mental health field have shown accuracy and efficiency in the diagnosis and treatment of depression (Laacke et al. 2021). On examining AI-driven technologies in relation to diagnosing mental disorders, it was found that AI showed significantly high levels of accuracy and sensitivity in detecting and diagnosing mental disorders (Alaa Abd-Alrazaq et al. 2022), thus showcasing its advantage for clinicians in terms or rapid accuracy and diagnosis. EAI and ML have been a recent attention in studies. The adoption of these technologies can help overcome some of the shortcomings of conventional screening approaches, as EAI and ML have the potential to increase the accuracy and reliability of depression detection (Joshi and Kanoongo 2022).

As a result, it is possible to see the overview of the present body of research on the use of AI-driven technologies to diagnose mental disorders and its support towards professionals. These technologies have the potential to lead to better diagnosis and treatment outcomes while also highlighting the most significant problems that need to be addressed.

10.7.1. *Implication*

– The study suggests practical applications for these self-learning chatbots, machine learning and mental health apps that are more individualized for the patient and has a fully objective view. Additionally, they help those who are hesitant to open up by giving them a foundation or safe environment where they can do so.

– The study discovered that mental healthcare delivered by AI-based care is faster and enables rapid diagnosis. Therefore, taking up less time and being a more time-effective therapy.

– There is an increase in the number of patients who need mental healthcare as the population grows. As a result, AI may assist with basic administrative tasks and various types of diagnosis and assessment, substantially simplifying the work of clinicians.

10.7.2. *Limitations*

– Few research had insufficient data since the publication was only partially accessible, which constrained the resources.

– The study did not explore AI about all disorders, and it was mainly narrowed down to mood disorders (i.e. depression, anxiety and bipolar disorder) and schizophrenia.

10.8. Suggestions for future studies

The following research directions are suggested for subsequent studies:

Future studies can research the combined effect of in-person mental healthcare provision along with AI-based and further compare it with individualized use of each one of them respectively.

Further research needs to be conducted on ethical implications related to AI-based intervention.

10.9. Conclusion

After reviewing 40 research papers, we found emerging themes in their findings. AI has an immense amount of potential and has shown promise in the field of mental healthcare. Preliminary technologies, such as mental healthcare applications and chatbots, have shown positive results, but there are no comprehensive guardrails on this technology yet. Moreover, it has been a valuable development for psychological professionals and has benefited users. Several ethical points of view have to be considered, and a comprehensive framework has to be formed around using AI for mental healthcare. Mental healthcare through AI, if left unsupervised, has the possibility of causing more harm than good. AI could give incorrect or harmful advice to patients or have interventions with them that are unsuitable for their particular issue. Therefore, detailed understandings, research and testing must be carried out before AI can become mainstream in mental healthcare.

10.10. Appendix

Author and year	Country	Design	Sample	Type of health care provision	Target Users	Objective	Ethics	Results
Mörch et al. (2020)	Canada	Checklist method	149 researchers	AI-based	Those who research, design and/or develop AI systems. Health practitioners with a background in mental health and computer scientists	Aid users in evaluating the informational resources available to them regarding potential ethical difficulties for their project or organization	Privacy and transparency, data security, health-related risks, informed consent	Provided a framework for ethical development, implementation, and evaluation for AI-based intervention Emphasized on the importance of ethical considerations in AI-based mental health intervention
Fiske, Henningsen and Buyx (2019)	Germany	Literature review	Research studies and academic literature on the topic of embodied AI in mental health care.	Embodied AI applications	Clients in need of dementia care and autistic disorder, sexual disorder	Patient privacy, informed consent, data security, and potential biases in the development of AI algorithms	Harm prevention, data ethics; lack of guidance on the development of AI applications	Highlighted the need for guidelines and regulations for the development and implementation of embodied AI in alignment with ethics and protecting patient safety
Fulmer et al. (2018)	UK	Randomized controlled trial	75	Computer-assisted therapy and conversational chatbot delivering cognitive behavioral therapy (CBT)	College students	Evaluate the viability and effectiveness of using Tess, an integrative psychological AI, to lessen college students' reported symptoms of anxiety and depression	To maintain participant privacy, all information, including usage, was de-identified and presented only as a mean	A statistically significant difference between group 1 and the control group, with group 1 reporting a substantial decrease in depressive symptoms as assessed by the PHQ-9 ($P = 0.03$) whereas the control group did not

Owusu et al. (2021)	Germany	Systematic review	n/a	AI applications in social media	Internet/social media users	The goal is to understand the content validity of algorithms for detecting depression screening tool based on AI on social media	User privacy, transparency, avoid stigmatization	Highlighted the advantages of using AI for depression screening and emphasized on the importance of these tools being clinically and ethically appropriate
Min LIM et al. (2021)	Singapore	A systematic review and meta-regression	Studies with a total of 1,263 participants receiving chatbot-delivered psychotherapy	Chatbot-delivered psychotherapy	Adults with depressive and anxiety symptoms	Efficacy of chatbot-delivered psychotherapy in reducing depressive symptoms in adults suffering from depression or anxiety	n/a	Chatbot-delivered psychotherapy was associated with reductions in depressive and anxiety symptoms The quality of evidence was found to be low, and more research is needed to establish this
Martinengo et al. (2022)	Singapore and UK	Content analysis	9 conventional agents (CAs)	Chatbot-delivered interventions	Individuals in need of self-management of depression	The structure, content, and user-customization of mental health CA conversations with users who were depressed or suicidal	n/a	Assessed CAs provided anonymous, compassionate and nonjudgmental interactions that are consistent with the research on in-person psychotherapy

Min LIM et al. (2021)	Singapore	A systematic review and meta-regression	Studies with a total of 1,263 participants receiving chatbot-delivered psychotherapy.	Chatbot-delivered psychotherapy	Adults with depressive and anxiety symptoms	Efficacy of chatbot-delivered psychotherapy in reducing depressive symptoms in adults suffering from depression or anxiety	n/a	Chatbot-delivered psychotherapy was associated with reductions in depressive and anxiety symptoms The quality of evidence was found to be low, and more research is needed to establish this
Wang et al. (2022)	South Korea	Study	76 eighth-grade students	Artificial intelligence robot Xiaoxin	Individuals in need of mental healthcare	Intervention effect of AI in the middle school students' one-to-one psychological intervention system, and ascertain whether middle school students have sufficient trust in AI machines	n/a	The use of AI-based emotional regulation and intervention system improved middle school students' emotional regulation and decreased negative emotions
Han et al. (2019)	South Korea and Italy	Research article	320 individuals	Structural MRI	Individuals in need of mental healthcare	Structural and functional magnetic resonance imaging (MRI) studies that, using various neuroimaging techniques, directly contrast UD and BD depression	n/a	Compared to UD, BD displayed less integrity in the posterior cingulum and the anterior part of the corpus callosum

Tennenhouse et al. (2020)	Canada	Research article	637 participants	Machine learning models	Individuals in need of mental healthcare	To predict depression and anxiety in people with immune-mediated inflammatory disease (IMID), look into the use of machine learning algorithms	Informed consent, privacy protection and transparency	ML models accurately predict depression and anxiety in individuals with IMID The models' accuracy is 78% and 79% respectively
Richter et al. (2021)	Israel	Research article	86 psychiatric patients and 25 participants with no psychiatric diagnosis	Machine learning	Individuals in need of mental healthcare (clinical anxiety and depression disorders)	Explains a novel diagnostic aid designed to distinguish between anxiety and depressive illnesses in a clinical sample	n/a	Along with the clinical interview, the cognitive battery can be used as a support system for mental diagnosis

10.11. References

Abd-Alrazaq, A.A., Alajlani, M., Alalwan, A.A., Bewick, B.M., Gardner, P., Househ, M. (2019). An overview of the features of chatbots in mental health: A scoping review. *International Journal of Medical Informatics*, 132, 103978. doi: 10.1016/j.ijmedinf.2019.103978.

Abd-Alrazaq, A.A., Alajlani, M., Alalwan, A.A., Bewick, B.M., Gardner, P., Househ, M. (2022). The performance of artificial intelligence-driven technologies in diagnosing mental disorders: An umbrella review. *npj Digital Medicine*, 5(1). doi: 10.1038/s41746-022-00631-8.

Akdeniz, E., Alp, F., Demirbaş, M., Akalın, B. (2022). Investigation of data types used in artificial intelligence approaches in psychiatry. *Uluslararası Sağlık Bilimleri ve Yönetimi Kongresi* [Preprint] [Online]. Available at: https://www.researchgate.net/publication/362668730_Investigation_of_Data_Types_Used_in_Artificial_Intelligence_Approaches_in_Psychiatry.

Baabdullah, A.M., Alalwan, A.A., Algharabat, R.S., Metri, B., Rana. N.P. (2022). Virtual agents and flow experience: An empirical examination of AI-powered chatbots. *Technological Forecasting and Social Change*, 181, 121772. doi: 10.1016/j.techfore.2022.121772.

Barnett, I., Torous, J., Staples, P., Sandoval, L., Keshavan, M., Onnela, J.-P. (2018). Relapse prediction in schizophrenia through digital phenotyping: A pilot study. *Neuropsychopharmacology*, 43(8), 1660–1666. doi: 10.1038/s41386-018-0030-z.

Blease, C., Kharko, A., Annoni, M., Gaab, J., Locher. C. (2021). Machine learning in clinical psychology and psychotherapy education: A mixed methods pilot survey of postgraduate students at a Swiss University. *Frontiers in Public Health*, 9. doi: 10.3389/fpubh.2021.623088.

Cecula, P., Yu, J., Dawoodbhoy, F.M., Delaney, J., Tan, J., Peacock, I., Cox, B. (2021). Applications of artificial intelligence to improve patient flow on mental health inpatient units – Narrative literature review. *Heliyon*, 7(4), e06626. doi: 10.1016/j.heliyon.2021.e06626.

Ćosić, K., Popović, S., Šarlija, M., Kesedžić, I., Gambiraža, M., Dropuljić, B., Mijić, I., Henigsberg, N., Jovanovic, T. (2021b). AI-based prediction and prevention of psychological and behavioral changes in ex-COVID-19 patients. *Frontiers in Psychology*, 12. doi: 10.3389/fpsyg.2021.782866.

D'Alfonso, S., Santesteban-Echarri, O., Rice, S., Wadley, G., Lederman, R., Miles, C., Gleeson, J., Alvarez-Jimenez, M. (2017). Artificial intelligence-assisted online social therapy for youth mental health. *Frontiers in Psychology*, 8. doi: 10.3389/fpsyg.2017.00796.

DelveInsight (2023). Artificial intelligence (AI) in mental health applications, benefits. DelveInsight Business Research [Online]. Available at: https://www.delveinsight.com/blog/artificial-intelligence-in-mental-health.

First, M.B. (2023b). Treatment of mental illness. MSD Manual, Consumer Version [Online]. Available at: https://www.msdmanuals.com/en-in/home/mental-health-disorders/overview-of-mental-health-care/treatment-of-mental-illness.

Fiske, A., Henningsen, P., Buyx, A. (2019). Your robot therapist will see you now: Ethical implications of embodied artificial intelligence in psychiatry, psychology, and psychotherapy. *Journal of Medical Internet Research*, 21(5), e13216. doi: 10.2196/13216.

Fulmer, R., Joerin, A., Gentile, B., Lakerink, L., Rauws, M. (2018). Using psychological artificial intelligence (Tess) to relieve symptoms of depression and anxiety: Randomized controlled trial. *JMIR Mental Health*, 5(4), e64. doi: 10.2196/mental.9782.

Gamble, A. (2020). Artificial intelligence and mobile apps for mental healthcare: A social informatics perspective. *Aslib Proceedings*, 72(4), 509–523. doi: 10.1108/ajim-11-2019-0316.

Gao, S., Calhoun, V.D., Sui, J. (2018b). Machine learning in major depression: From classification to treatment outcome prediction. *CNS Neuroscience and Therapeutics*, 24(11), 1037–1052. doi: 10.1111/cns.13048.

Gerke, S., Minssen, T., Cohen, G. (2020). Ethical and legal challenges of artificial intelligence-driven healthcare. In *Artificial Intelligence in Healthcare*, Bohr, A. and Memarzadeh, K. (eds). Academic Press, Cambridge, MA. doi: 10.1016/B978-0-12-818438-7.00012-5.

Grainger, R. and Sikka, R. (2020). Ethical considerations in the use of artificial intelligence in mental health care. *Current Opinion in Psychiatry*, 33(3), 236–240.

Han, K.-M., De Berardis, D., Fornaro, M., Kim. Y.-K. (2019). Differentiating between bipolar and unipolar depression in functional and structural MRI studies. *Progress in Neuropsychopharmacology and Biological Psychiatry*, 91, 20–27. doi: 10.1016/j.pnpbp.2018.03.022.

Hatch, S.L., Harvey, S.B., Maughan, B. (2010). A developmental-contextual approach to understanding mental health and well-being in early adulthood. *Social Science and Medicine*, 70(2), 261–268. doi: 10.1016/j.socscimed.2009.10.005.

Hueniken, K., Somé, N.H., Abdelhack, M., Taylor, G., Marshall, T.E., Wickens, C.M., Hamilton, H.A., Wells, S., Felsky, D. (2021). Machine learning-based predictive modeling of anxiety and depressive symptoms during 8 months of the Covid-19 global pandemic: Repeated cross-sectional survey study. *JMIR Mental Health*, 8(11), e32876. doi: 10.2196/32876.

IEEE (2022). Improving mental health with machine learning. *IEEE Innovation at Work* [Online]. Available at: https://innovationatwork.ieee.org/improving-mental-health-with-machine-learning/#:~:text=With%20the%20help%20of%20AI,determine%20a%20patient's%20optimal%20treatment.

IGI Global (n.d.). What is deep learning (DL) [Online]. Available at: https://www.igi-global.com/dictionary/deep-learning-in-instructional-analysis-design-development-implementation-and-evaluation-addie/59656.

Jacobson, N.C. and Nemesure, M.D. (2021). Using artificial intelligence to predict change in depression and anxiety symptoms in a digital intervention: Evidence from a transdiagnostic randomized controlled trial. *Psychiatry Research: Neuroimaging*, 295, 113618. doi: 10.1016/j.psychres.2020.113618.

Joshi, M.B. and Kanoongo, N. (2022). Depression detection using emotional artificial intelligence and machine learning: A closer review. *Materials Today: Proceedings*, 58, 217–226. doi: 10.1016/j.matpr.2022.01.467.

Kazdin, A.E. and Blase, S.L. (2011). Rebooting psychotherapy research and practice to reduce the burden of mental illness. *Perspectives on Psychological Science*, 6(1), 21–37. doi: 10.1177/1745691610393527.

Keyes, C.L.M. (2002). The mental health continuum: From languishing to flourishing in life. *Journal of Health and Social Behavior*, 43(2), 207. doi: 10.2307/3090197.

Klos, M.C., Escoredo, M., Joerin, A., Lemos, V.N., Rauws, M., Bunge, E.L. (2021). Artificial intelligence-based chatbot for anxiety and depression in university students: Pilot randomized controlled trial. *JMIR Formative Research*, 5(8), e20678. doi: 10.2196/20678.

Laacke, S., Mueller, R., Schomerus, G., Salloch. S. (2021). Artificial intelligence, social media and depression. A new concept of health-related digital autonomy. *American Journal of Bioethics*, 21(7), 4–20. doi: 10.1080/15265161.2020.1863515.

Lavrentyeva, Y. (2023b). The big promise AI holds for mental health. ITRex [Online]. Available at: https://itrexgroup.com/blog/ai-mental-health-examples-trends/.

Lee, E., Torous, J., De Choudhury, M., Depp, C.A., Graham, S., Kim, H., Paulus, M.P., Krystal, J.H., Jeste, D.V. (2021). Artificial intelligence for mental health care: Clinical applications, barriers, facilitators, and artificial wisdom. *Biological Psychiatry: Cognitive Neuroscience and Neuroimaging*, 6(9), 856–864. doi: 10.1016/j.bpsc.2021.02.001.

Lim, S.T., Shiau, C.W.C., Cheng, L.J., Lau, Y. (2022). Chatbot-delivered psychotherapy for adults with depressive and anxiety symptoms: A systematic review and meta-regression. *Behavior Therapy*, 53(2), 334–347. doi: 10.1016/j.beth.2021.09.007.

Liu, H., Peng, H., Song, X., Xu, C., Zhang, M. (2022). Using AI chatbots to provide self-help depression interventions for university students: A randomized trial of effectiveness. *Internet Interventions*, 27, 100495. doi: 10.1016/j.invent.2022.100495.

Mann, M., Kumar, C., Zeng, W.F., Strauss, M.T. (2021). Artificial intelligence for proteomics and biomarker discovery. *Cell Systems*, 12(8), 759–770.

Martinengo, L., Lum, E., Car, J. (2022). Evaluation of chatbot-delivered interventions for self-management of depression: Content analysis. *Journal of Affective Disorders*, 319, 598–607. doi: 10.1016/j.jad.2022.09.028.

Martinez-Martin, N. and Kreitmair, K.V. (2018). Ethical issues for direct-to-consumer digital psychotherapy apps: Addressing accountability, data protection, and consent. *JMIR Mental Health*, 5(2), e32. doi: 10.2196/mental.9423.

Mehta, A., Niles, A.N., Vargas, J.H., Marafon, T., Couto, D.D., Gross, J.J. (2021). Acceptability and effectiveness of artificial intelligence therapy for anxiety and depression (Youper): Longitudinal observational study. *Journal of Medical Internet Research*, 23(6), e26771. doi: 10.2196/26771.

Merchant, S. (2021). These chatbots are helping with mental health right now. AIM [Online]. Available at: https://www.aimblog.io/2021/03/02/these-chatbots-are-helping-with-mental-health-right-now/.

Milne-Ives, M., Selby, E., Inkster, B., Lam, C., Meinert, E. (2022). Artificial intelligence and machine learning in mobile apps for mental health: A scoping review. *PLOS Digital Health*, 1(8), e0000079. doi: 10.1371/journal.pdig.0000079.

Monteith, S., Glenn, T., Geddes, J., Whybrow, P.C., Bauer, M. (2022). Commercial use of emotion artificial intelligence (AI): Implications for psychiatry. *Current Psychiatry Reports*, 24(3), 203–211. doi: 10.1007/s11920-022-01330-7.

Mörch, C.-M., Gupta, A., Mishara, B.L. (2020). Canada protocol: An ethical checklist for the use of artificial intelligence in suicide prevention and mental health. *Artificial Intelligence in Medicine*, 108, 101934. doi: 10.1016/j.artmed.2020.101934.

Naqishbandi, T., Syed, M., Aijaz, D., Zameer, G. (2021b). Artificial intelligence in mental healthcare analytics: Opportunities, future risks, and regulations. In *4th International Education and Innovative Sciences Symposium* [Online]. Available at: https://www.researchgate.net/publication/356714991_ARTIFICIAL_INTELLIGENCE_IN_MENTAL_HEALTHCARE_ANALYTICS_OPPORTUNITIES_FUTURE_RISKS_AND_REGULATIONS.

NHS (n.d.) Overview – Cognitive behavioral therapy (CBT) [Online]. Available at: https://www.nhs.uk/mental-health/talking-therapies-medicine-treatments/talking-therapies-and-counselling/cognitive-behavioral-therapy-cbt/overview/#:~:text=Cognitive%20behavioral%20therapy%20(CBT)%20is.

Nunez, J.J., Nguyen, T.T., Zhou, Y., Cao, B., Ng, R.T., Chen, J., Frey, B.N., Milev, R., Müller, D.J., Rotzinger, S. et al. (2021). Replication of machine learning methods to predict treatment outcome with antidepressant medications in patients with major depressive disorder from STAR*D and CAN-BIND-1. *PLOS ONE*, 16(6), e0253023. doi: 10.1371/journal.pone.0253023.

Owusu, P.N., Reininghaus, U., Koppe, G., Dankwa-Mullan, I., Bärnighausen, T. (2021). Artificial intelligence applications in social media for depression screening: A systematic review protocol for content validity processes. *PLOS ONE*, 16(11), e0259499. doi: 10.1371/journal.pone.0259499.

Parvez, N. (2022). Can machine learning be used to improve mental health? Analytics Insight [Online]. Available at: https://www.analyticsinsight.net/can-machine-learning-be-used-to-improve-mental-health/.

Pereira, S., Cavaco, A., Ferreira, C. (2021). The potential of artificial intelligence in mental health: A review of current evidence. *Advances in Intelligent Systems and Computing*, 1175, 193–204. doi: 10.1007/978-3-030-71538-8_19.

Radcliffe Publishing and Wonca (2008). What is primary care mental health? WHO and Wonca Working Party on Mental Health. *Ment. Health Fam. Med.*, 5(1), 9–13 [Online]. Available at: https://www.ncbi.nlm.nih.gov/pmc/articles/PMC2777553/.

Rajpurkar, P., Yang, J., Dass, N., Vale, V., Keller, A.S., Irvin, J., Taylor, Z., Basu, S., Ng, A., Williams, L.M. (2020). Evaluation of a machine learning model based on pretreatment symptoms and electroencephalographic features to predict outcomes of antidepressant treatment in adults with depression. *JAMA Network Open*, 3(6), e206653. doi: 10.1001/jamanetworkopen.2020.6653.

Richter, T., Fishbain, B., Fruchter, E., Richter-Levin, G., Okon-Singer, H. (2021). Machine learning-based diagnosis support system for differentiating between clinical anxiety and depression disorders. *Journal of Psychiatric Research*, 141, 199–205. doi: 10.1016/j.jpsychires.2021.06.044.

Rozek, D.C., Andres, W.C., Smith, N.B., Leifker, F.R., Arne, K., Jennings, G., Dartnell, N., Bryan, C.J., Rudd. M.D. (2020b). Using machine learning to predict suicide attempts in military personnel. *Psychiatry Research: Neuroimaging*, 294, 113515. doi: 10.1016/j.psychres.2020.113515.

SAMHSA (n.d.). What is mental health? [Online]. Available at: https://www.mentalhealth.gov/basics/what-is-mental-health.

Shatte, A., Hutchinson, D., Teague, S. (2019b). Machine learning in mental health: A scoping review of methods and applications. *Psychological Medicine*, 49(09), 1426–1448. doi: 10.1017/s0033291719000151.

Sutton, J. (2023). Artificial intelligence in psychology: 9 examples and apps. PositivePsychology.com [Online]. Available at: https://positivepsychology.com/artificial-intelligence-in-psychology/.

Tennenhouse, L.G., Marrie, R.A., Bernstein, C.N., Lix, L.M. (2020). Machine-learning models for depression and anxiety in individuals with immune-mediated inflammatory disease. *Journal of Psychosomatic Research*, 134, 110126. doi: 10.1016/j.jpsychores.2020.110126.

Thermolia, C.H., Bei, E.S., Petrakis, E.G.M. (2015). AI-care: A clinical decision support system with application in bipolar disorder. *European Psychiatry*, 30, 1905. doi: 10.1016/s0924-9338(15)31457-7.

Thieme, A., Belgrave, D., Doherty, G. (2020). Machine learning in mental health. *ACM Transactions on Computer-Human Interaction*, 27(5), 1–53. doi: 10.1145/3398069.

Torous, J., Bucci, S., Bell, I., Kessing, L.V., Faurholt-Jepsen, M., Whelan, P., Carvalho, A.F., Keshavan, M.S., Linardon, J., Firth, J. (2021). The growing field of digital psychiatry: Current evidence and the future of apps, social media, chatbots, and virtual reality. *World Psychiatry*, 20(3), 318–335. doi: 10.1002/wps.20883.

Tymofiyeva, O., Yuan, J.P., Huang, C.-Yu., Connolly, C.G., Blom, E.H., Xu, D., Yang, T.T. (2019). Application of machine learning to structural connectome to predict symptom reduction in depressed adolescents with cognitive behavioral therapy (CBT). *NeuroImage: Clinical*, 23, 101914. doi: 10.1016/j.nicl.2019.101914.

Venturi, D. (2021). How AI is changing mental health care – David Venturi. Medium, 2 January [Online]. Available at: https://davidventuri.medium.com/how-ai-is-revolutionizing-mental-health-care-a7cec436a1ce.

Villongco, C.T. and Khan, F.H. (2020). 'Sorry I Didn't Hear You.'. The ethics of voice computing and AI in high risk mental health populations. *AJOB Neuroscience*. doi: 10.1080/21507740.2020.1740355.

Wang, E., Chang. W.L., Shen, J., Bian, Q., Huang, P., Lai, X., Chang, T.Y., Shaoying, H., Ziyue, Z., Wang, Z. et al. (2022). Effect of artificial intelligence on one-to-one emotional regulation and psychological intervention system of middle school students. *International Journal of Neuropsychopharmacology*, 25(Supplement 1), A62–A63. doi: 10.1093/ijnp/pyac032.086.

Watts, D., Pulice, R.F., Reilly, J., Brunoni, A.R., Kapczinski, F., Passos, I.C. (2022). Predicting treatment response using EEG in major depressive disorder: A machine-learning meta-analysis. *Translational Psychiatry*, 12(1). doi: 10.1038/s41398-022-02064-z.

World Economic Forum (2021). 4 ways artificial intelligence is improving mental health therapy [Online]. Available at: https://www.weforum.org/agenda/2021/12/ai-mental-health-cbt-therapy/.

Yang, F., Xie, J., Zhong, Z.-B. (2021). The application prospects of artificial intelligence in the field of mental health and hygiene. *Edpsciences*, 275, 03042. doi: 10.1051/e3sconf/202127503042.

Zhang, X., Wang, R., Sharma, A., Deverajan, G.G. (2021). Artificial intelligence in cognitive psychology – Influence of literature based on artificial intelligence on children's mental disorders. *Aggression and Violent Behavior*, 101590. doi: 10.1016/j.avb.2021.101590.

Zhang, T., Schoene, A.M., Ji, S., Ananiadou, S. (2022). Natural language processing applied to mental illness detection: A narrative review. *npj Digital Medicine*, 5(1). doi: 10.1038/s41746-022-00589-7.

11

Unleashing the Future: Exploring the Transformative Potential of 5G Technology in Healthcare

The emergence of 5G technology marks a significant advancement in the realm of wireless communication and connectivity. As the fifth generation of wireless technology, 5G introduces unprecedented speed, capacity and responsiveness, poised to reshape industries and redefine user experiences. This abstract encapsulates the essence of 5G by highlighting its transformative potential. From blazing data speeds and real-time applications to mass device connectivity through the Internet of Things (IoT), 5G unlocks a world of possibilities. However, its deployment necessitates infrastructure enhancements and raises discussions about privacy, security and health considerations. The abstract underscores the need for a balanced approach to harnessing 5G's benefits while addressing its challenges. In the grand scheme of technological evolution, 5G's arrival stands as a pivotal milestone with far-reaching implications across society, business and innovation.

11.1. Introduction to 5G technology

In the landscape of modern communication and connectivity, 5G technology stands as a groundbreaking milestone poised to redefine the way we connect, communicate and interact with the digital world. As the fifth generation of wireless technology, 5G represents a leap forward in terms of speed, capacity, responsiveness and the possibilities it unlocks for a wide range of industries and applications. With its potential to revolutionize everything from mobile data usage to the Internet of

Chapter written by Varalakshmi DANDU.
For a color version of all the figures in this chapter, see www.iste.co.uk/pradhan/cognitivecomputing.zip.

Things (IoT) and beyond, 5G is not only an upgrade to previous cellular generations but also a technological shift that holds the power to shape the future of global communication and innovation.

At its core, 5G technology promises to deliver data speeds and capabilities that were once deemed unimaginable. It capitalizes on advancements in wireless infrastructure, spectrum utilization and signal processing to achieve data transfer rates up to 100 times faster than its predecessor, 4G LTE. This unparalleled speed not only enables seamless streaming of high-definition content but also paves the way for real-time applications that demand instant responsiveness, such as augmented reality, virtual reality and telemedicine.

Beyond its speed, 5G introduces a paradigm shift in connectivity through its ability to handle an exponentially greater number of devices simultaneously. This mass device connectivity is vital for the expansion of the IoT, where everyday objects and machines communicate and share data to enhance efficiency and convenience across various sectors. From smart cities and autonomous vehicles to industrial automation and healthcare applications, the ability of 5G to facilitate interconnectivity on a massive scale lays the foundation for a more intelligent and interconnected world.

However, the journey to fully realizing the potential of 5G is not without its challenges. The deployment of 5G requires a comprehensive infrastructure overhaul, including the installation of small cells, advanced antennas and fiber-optic networks to support the increased demand for faster and more reliable connectivity. Furthermore, as 5G operates on higher-frequency bands, it faces coverage limitations and potential signal blockage, particularly in dense urban environments or remote areas.

While 5G offers a plethora of advantages, it also raises important discussions about privacy, security and potential health concerns due to increased electromagnetic radiation exposure. Striking a balance between reaping the benefits of advanced connectivity and addressing these considerations is crucial for the responsible and effective integration of 5G technology into our lives.

5G technology represents a pivotal moment in the evolution of wireless communication. With its promise of lightning-fast speeds, massive device connectivity and transformative applications, 5G has the potential to reshape industries, elevate consumer experiences and foster innovation on a global scale. As this technology continues to unfold, its impacts on society, business and technology will undoubtedly be profound, ushering in a new era of connectivity and possibilities.

11.2. Definition of 5G

5G, or the fifth generation of wireless technology, is the latest evolution in telecommunications standards. It is designed to provide significantly faster data speeds, lower latency and the ability to connect a massive number of devices simultaneously, paving the way for new applications and services.

11.3. History of 5G evolution

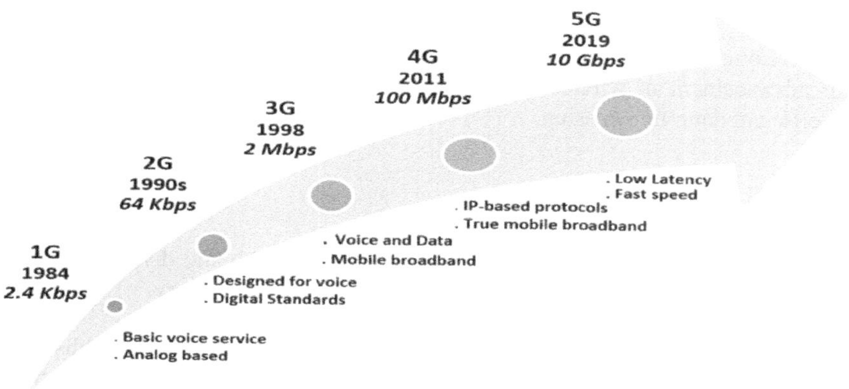

Figure 11.1. *Evolution of 5G. Source: https://link.springer.com/article/10.1007/s12652-020-02521-x*

The evolution of 5G technology has been a multi-decade process, marked by various advancements in wireless communication standards. The following sections present a brief history of the key milestones leading up to the development and deployment of 5G.

11.3.1. *1G to 3G (1980s–2000s)*

1G (first generation): introduced in the early 1980s, 1G provided analog voice communication. It was the first step towards wireless mobility, but it had limited capacity and security.

2G (second generation): rolled out in the 1990s, 2G brought digital communication and introduced features like text messaging (SMS) and basic data services.

3G (third generation): emerged in the early 2000s, 3G provided higher data speeds and enabled mobile Internet access, paving the way for services such as video calling and mobile web browsing.

11.3.2. *4G and LTE (late 2000s–early 2010s)*

4G (fourth generation): 4G technology, introduced around 2009, significantly improved data speeds, offering high-definition video streaming and better mobile Internet experiences.

LTE (Long-Term Evolution): often used interchangeably with 4G, LTE was a major advancement in wireless technology, providing a foundation for faster and more efficient data transmission.

11.3.3. *The path to 5G (2010s)*

2012–2014: the groundwork for 5G began with research and discussions on the technical requirements of the next generation of wireless technology.

2015: the International Telecommunication Union-Radio (ITU-R) established the broad goals and technical criteria for 5G networks, setting the stage for its development.

11.3.4. *Key milestones towards 5G (2016–2019)*

2016: trials and experiments of early 5G technologies began, focusing on concepts like millimeter-wave frequencies and massive MIMO (Multiple-Input Multiple-Output) for higher data rates and capacity.

2017: the first official 5G New Radio (NR) standard was announced by the 3rd Generation Partnership Project (3GPP), a collaborative organization responsible for defining mobile communication standards.

2018: initial 5G deployments took place in a few cities, primarily targeting fixed wireless access (FWA) and enhanced mobile broadband.

2019: commercial 5G networks were launched in several countries, bringing faster speeds and lower latency to users in select areas.

11.3.5. *5G deployment and expansion (2020s)*

2020–2021: 5G adoption continued to grow globally, with more countries rolling out commercial networks and expanding coverage. The Covid-19 pandemic highlighted the importance of robust connectivity.

2022 and beyond: 5G technology is expected to continue evolving, with increasing coverage, improved reliability and the realization of advanced use cases such as autonomous vehicles, smart cities and industrial automation.

Throughout this evolution, the telecommunications industry, regulatory bodies and technology developers have collaborated to push the boundaries of wireless communication. 5G represents a significant leap forward in terms of speed, capacity and capabilities, with the potential to transform industries and enable a new era of connected devices and services.

5G, the fifth-generation mobility networking architecture, has the potential to revolutionize how we live, what we do, how we communicate and how society and the industry operates.

In 5G, an ecosystem that will connect virtually everyone and everything, including machines, objects and devices is being built.

5G bridges the digital barrier by providing not only high-speed connectivity but also higher reliability, higher network capacity and low latency.

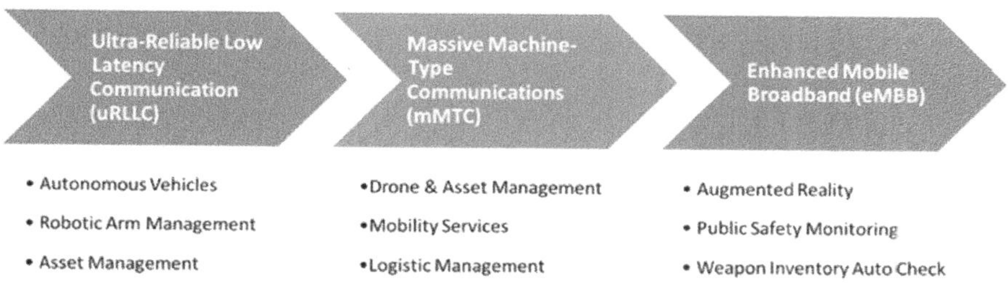

Figure 11.2. *Applications of the 5G network. Source: https://stl.tech/blog/the-evolution-of-5g-and-its-use-cases*

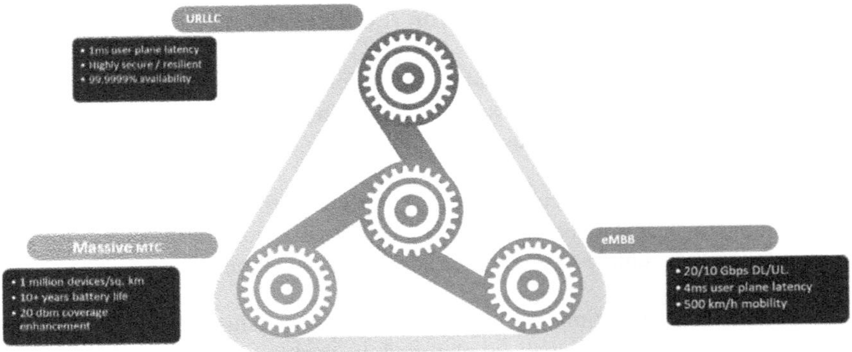
URLLC
• 1ms user plane latency
• Highly secure / resilient
• 99.9999% availability
Massive MTC
• 1 million devices/sq. km
• 10+ years battery life
• 20 dbm coverage enhancement
eMBB
• 20/10 Gbps DL/UL
• 4ms user plane latency
• 500 km/h mobility

Figure 11.3. *Major proponents of a digital network. Source: https://stl.tech/blog/the-evolution-of-5g-and-its-use-cases*

Speed, capacity, latency, coverage and reliability are the major proponents of a digital network. 5G networks infuse substantial improvements over these parameters vis-a-vis their predecessor networks.

The following sections present some of the highlights of 5G technology that we can look forward to in the real-world use cases. Figure 11.4 presents a comparative analysis of some of the parameters between 4G and 5G.

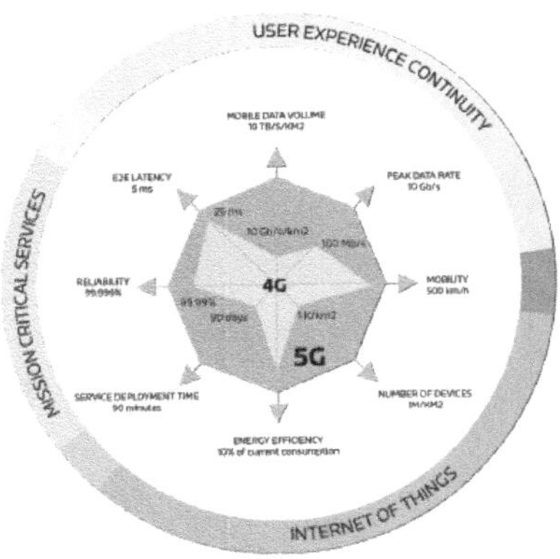

Figure 11.4. *Comparative analysis of 4G and 5G. Source: https://stl.tech/blog/the-evolution-of-5g-and-its-use-cases*

11.4. 5G bands

Spectrum plays a critical role in realizing the full extent of new capabilities in 5G. The full socio-economic impact of 5G depends on access to a variety of spectrum resources.

The spectrum bands (range of frequencies) used for 5G are categorized into two major categories (frequency range): FR1 and FR2, which are further divided into smaller bands. Table 11.1 gives an insight into the FR1 and FR2 bands used extensively in 5G.

Parameter	Low bands (FR1)	Mid-bands (FR1)	High bands (FR2: mmWave)
Frequency range	Sub 1 GHz	1–7 GHz	24–52 GHz
Major 5G bands in India	n5, n8, n20, n28	n1, n3, n40, n41, n77, n78	n257, n258
Coverage	Wide coverage area	High-density coverage area	Very high-density coverage area
Capacity	Limited capacity	High capacity	Ultra-high capacity
Carrier BW	Up to 100 MHz	Up to 400 MHz	
Max. carriers	8		

Table 11.1. *Spectrum bands of 5G. Source: https://stl.tech/blog/the-evolution-of-5g-and-its-use-cases*

i) Low-frequency FR1 bands: these bands are sub-1 GHz FR1 bands used for wide coverage areas but come with the limitation of limited carrier capacity. These are rarely used for high capacity requirements due to the limited channel bandwidth.

ii) Mid-frequency FR1 bands: these bands range from 1 GHz to 7 GHz and are being used for 5G extensively. This is attributed to their capacity and coverage equilibrium, which is ideal for 5G services. Mid bands play a key role in meeting the demand for mobile data services. New mobile broadband use cases such as enhanced mobile broadband, fixed wireless access, IoT and Industry 4.0 depend on the mid-band spectrum. As a result of these use cases, mobile services will have a greater impact on society and the economy than ever before. To date, the mid-band spectrum has been the most commonly used around the globe to launch 5G networks. This band will be the highest revenue earner as it provides high capacity with higher coverage.

iii) Millimeter wave FR2 bands: the FR2 bands range from 7 GHz to 100 GHz. The most relevant sub-range in the FR2 bands is 24 GHz–52 GHz and is commonly referred to as the mm Wave band. This band is best suited for very high-density areas as it provides very high capacity, which comes with the limitation of smaller coverage areas.

11.5. 5G use cases and spectrum band relevance

5G use cases are suitable for different frequency bands due to different requirements in terms of bandwidth, latency and other performance metrics. The applicability of different use cases in reference to the frequency bands is shown in Table 11.2.

Use case	Low bands	Mid-bands	mmWave bands
eMBB	10%	80%	10%
FWA	10%	60%	30%
MIoT	40%	60%	0%
URLLC	0%	40%	60%

Table 11.2. *5G use cases and spectrum band relevance. Source: https://stl.tech/blog/the-evolution-of-5g-and-its-use-cases*

11.6. 5G for industries

Technology has always been a solution to the industry's problem and is hence influential in the growth of the industries.

Emergent technologies such as the Internet of Things (IoT), artificial intelligence (AI), computer vision, drone/anti-drone technology, robotics, augmented reality (AR), virtual reality, parallel reality and quantum computing are revolutionizing different industries.

The arrival of 5G can unlock the positive impact of these technologies, thereby facilitating remote surveillance in homeland security and defense, remote healthcare, precision agriculture, safer transportation and digitized logistics.

Distribution and benefits	Enhanced mobile broadband (eMBB)	Fixed wireless access (FWA)	Massive IoT (MIoT)	Ultra-reliable, low-latency communication (URLLC)
Distribution	42%	32%	16%	10%
Benefits	Connected vehicles Smart wearables Virtual and augmented reality	High-speed broadband in sub-urban/ rural areas	Collaborative robots/complex automation Remote object manipulation	Connected vehicles Collaborative robots/complex automation Remote object manipulation

Table 11.3. *Benefits of mid-band 5G services. Source: https://stl.tech/blog/the-evolution-of-5g-and-its-use-cases*

11.7. Importance

The importance of 5G (fifth generation) technology lies in its potential to transform various industries, enhance user experiences and pave the way for innovative applications that were previously impractical or impossible. Here are some key aspects highlighting the significance of 5G.

11.7.1. *Faster data speeds*

5G offers significantly faster data transfer rates compared to previous generations. This speed boost enhances the overall user experience by allowing quicker downloads, seamless streaming of high-definition content and smoother online interactions.

11.7.2. *Ultra-low latency*

The reduced latency in 5G networks enables real-time communication, making applications like remote surgery, online gaming and industrial automation feasible. This is crucial for tasks that require instantaneous responses.

11.7.3. *Massive device connectivity*

5G networks can support a massive number of devices simultaneously. This is vital for the proliferation of the Internet of Things (IoT), where billions of interconnected devices can communicate efficiently and share data without overloading the network.

11.7.4. *Industrial automation and IoT*

5G's capabilities are well suited for industrial automation and IoT applications. It enables real-time monitoring and control of machinery, improving efficiency and reducing downtime in manufacturing and other industries.

11.7.5. *Healthcare advancements*

In the healthcare sector, 5G facilitates remote patient monitoring, telemedicine and even remote surgeries. Its low latency and high bandwidth enable medical professionals to collaborate and provide timely care regardless of geographical distances.

11.7.6. *Autonomous vehicles*

5G technology plays a crucial role in enabling connected and autonomous vehicles. Its low latency and reliable communication enable real-time vehicle-to-vehicle and vehicle-to-infrastructure communication, enhancing road safety and traffic management.

11.7.7. *Smart cities*

5G supports the development of smart cities by enabling efficient management of utilities, transportation systems and public services through interconnected sensors and devices. This can lead to reduced energy consumption, improved traffic flow and enhanced citizen services.

11.7.8. *Remote work and education*

The Covid-19 pandemic highlighted the importance of reliable and fast Internet connectivity for remote work and online education. 5G offers the potential for more stable connections and improved remote collaboration experiences.

11.7.9. *Entertainment and media*

With 5G, immersive experiences such as augmented reality (AR) and virtual reality (VR) become more accessible due to higher speeds and reduced latency. This enhances entertainment options and opens doors for new forms of content creation.

11.7.10. *Economic growth and innovation*

The deployment of 5G networks drives technological innovation and economic growth. It encourages businesses to develop new products, services and business models that leverage the capabilities of 5G, creating new job opportunities and revenue streams.

11.7.11. *Global competitiveness*

Countries and regions that lead in 5G deployment gain a competitive advantage in technology and innovation. Being at the forefront of 5G adoption can attract investment, foster research and position nations as leaders in the digital economy.

5G technology is not only about faster smartphones, but also a catalyst for transformative change across industries and society as a whole. Its high speeds, low latency and massive connectivity open up a world of possibilities, enabling innovative applications that can reshape how we live, work and interact with the world around us.

11.8. Key features of 5G

5G technology introduces several key features that set it apart from previous generations of wireless communication. These features enable enhanced performance, connectivity and support for a wide range of applications. Here are the prominent features of 5G:

– Faster data speeds: 5G offers substantially higher data transfer rates compared to previous generations. It can provide peak speeds of up to 20 gigabits per second (Gbps), allowing for ultra-fast downloads, uploads and streaming.

– Ultra-low latency: latency refers to the time it takes for data to travel from the sender to the receiver. 5G achieves extremely low latency levels, potentially as low as 1 millisecond. This near-instantaneous response is crucial for real-time applications such as remote surgery, online gaming and autonomous vehicles.

– Massive device connectivity: 5G is designed to support a massive number of devices per unit area. This is particularly important for the growing Internet of Things (IoT) ecosystem, where billions of interconnected devices, sensors and machines need to communicate simultaneously.

– Enhanced network capacity: the increased bandwidth and efficient use of frequency spectrum in 5G networks enable them to handle more users and devices concurrently without significant drops in performance. This is especially valuable in densely populated areas and during events where network congestion is common.

– Network slicing: 5G introduces the concept of network slicing, which allows a single physical network infrastructure to be divided into multiple virtual networks. Each slice can be optimized for specific use cases, ensuring that the network resources are allocated efficiently based on the requirements of different applications.

– Improved energy efficiency: 5G is designed with energy efficiency in mind. It includes technologies like advanced sleep modes and more efficient use of resources, which not only help to extend the battery life of devices but also contribute to reducing the environmental impact of network operations.

– Multi-gigabit throughput: 5G supports multi-gigabit data rates, enabling seamless high-definition and 4K video streaming, augmented and virtual reality experiences and other data-intensive applications.

– Beamforming and massive MIMO: 5G uses advanced antenna technologies such as beamforming and massive multiple-input multiple-output (MIMO) to direct signals precisely towards devices, improving signal strength, coverage and overall network efficiency.

– Improved security: while not solely a feature of 5G, security enhancements are integrated into 5G networks to address evolving cybersecurity threats. This includes stronger encryption protocols and authentication mechanisms.

– Enhanced location accuracy: 5G networks provide more accurate location data, which is vital for applications like emergency services, asset tracking and location-based services.

– Augmented reality (AR) and virtual reality (VR): the combination of high data speeds and low latency in 5G makes it well suited for immersive AR and VR experiences, enabling applications such as virtual meetings, remote training and interactive entertainment.

– Acceleration in speed: every advancement in wireless network technology has brought about a substantial boost in speed, and the advantages of 5G – referred to as the fifth generation of cellular network technology – will far surpass the capabilities of 4G LTE. Envisioned speeds of up to 10 Gbps translate to a remarkable 100-fold increase when compared to 4G. In practical terms, the speed enhancements from 4G to 5G will open up thrilling possibilities for consumers. The time it takes to download a high-resolution movie at peak speeds will shrink from seven minutes to a mere six seconds. Such time savings could enable individuals to obtain the latest movie hit before the flight attendant requests for phones be switched onto airplane mode. Once carriers fully implement the features of 5G, both consumers and businesses may begin to consider 5G networks as robust alternatives for rapid broadband connections.

– Reduced latency: latency signifies the duration a signal needs to travel from its source to its destination and back again. A consistent objective for each evolution of wireless technology has been to minimize latency. Upcoming 5G networks will exhibit even lower latency than 4G LTE, with data's round-trip transmission taking less than five milliseconds.

5G latency will surpass human visual processing speed, enabling real-time remote device control. Human reaction time will become the limiting factor for remote applications using 5G and the Internet of Things (IoT). Many new applications will involve machine-to-machine communication, unrestricted by human responsiveness. While agriculture, manufacturing and logistics will all gain from reduced latency, gamers are also eagerly anticipating the advent of 5G. The blend of high speed and minimal delay is tailor-made for applications in virtual reality (VR) and augmented reality (AR), which are likely to gain immense popularity as connectivity advancements offer a seamless, immersive experience.

– Enhanced capacity: although speed is exhilarating, a pertinent question is how 5G will support the expansion of business technology initiatives. 5G will offer up to 1,000 times greater capacity than 4G, creating fertile ground for the development of IoT. 5G and IoT are an ideal pairing, set to redefine the usage of wireless networks and the Internet on the whole. With the ability to seamlessly connect hundreds or thousands of devices, new applications and scenarios for cities, factories, farms, schools and residences will flourish. Picture 5G use cases involve thousands of sensors on numerous machines that automate supply chain management, ensuring timely material delivery and using predictive maintenance to minimize work disruptions. Smart homes and cities will also witness a significant leap in the era of 5G. With more connected devices than ever, AI will extend its reach through edge computing. From personalized energy-saving suggestions in households that maximize environmental impact to adaptive traffic lights based on traffic flow, 5G applications leveraging added network capacity will affect nearly everyone. From industrial automation to smart city traffic management, the augmented network capacity of 5G will impact a wide range of domains.

– Increased bandwidth: the conjunction of augmented speed and network capacity on 5G networks opens up the potential for transmitting larger data volumes than was ever feasible with 4G LTE networks. 5G networks have a distinct architecture from traditional 4G networks, enabling better network traffic optimization and seamless management of usage spikes. Crowded arenas and other venues have grappled with offering consistent connectivity to large audiences, but 5G could enable sports enthusiasts to stream their experiences from any spot in the stadium. For businesses, the influence of enhanced bandwidth will reverberate across numerous departments and divisions in the form of Big Data. Currently, companies receive an influx of information from customers, suppliers and teams that surpasses their processing and analytical capabilities. With 5G connectivity and Big Data analytics, these businesses can transform substantial data volumes into actionable insights.

– Availability and coverage: while consumers and businesses are eager to embrace the advantages of 5G, its coverage remains limited. Presently, major US cellular carriers are deploying 5G networks in major cities as they prepare for broader rollouts.

11.9. Intel 5G technologies and solutions

Realizing the full potential of 5G hinges on having a network can support next-generation capabilities and features. As a frontrunner in network solutions, Intel plays a pivotal role in the global 5G rollout's structure and organization. Intel's 5G technologies will fuel tomorrow's 5G experiences, ranging from edge devices collecting field data to network servers optimized for workloads, powered by Intel® Xeon® Scalable processors. Intel is committed to maximizing 5G's potential across its entire spectrum of applications and use cases, spanning from homes to workplaces and beyond. These features collectively make 5G a transformative technology that not only improves mobile communication but also opens up possibilities for innovative applications across various industries, from healthcare and transportation to manufacturing and entertainment. The adoption of 5G technology involves a multi-step process that includes infrastructure development, device compatibility, network deployment and the exploration of new use cases. Here is a breakdown of how 5G is adopted:

– Infrastructure development: telecommunication companies need to invest in building the necessary infrastructure to support 5G networks. This involves upgrading existing cell towers, installing new small cells in densely populated areas and ensuring adequate coverage to provide the promised high speeds and low latency.

– Device compatibility: manufacturers need to produce devices that are compatible with 5G technology. This includes smartphones, tablets, laptops, Internet of Things (IoT) devices and more. These devices need to have the necessary hardware and software components to communicate over 5G networks.

– Network deployment: the deployment of 5G networks is typically done in phases:

- initial trials: telecommunication providers conduct small-scale trials to test the new technology, optimize performance and identify potential challenges;

- limited rollouts: 5G is initially deployed in specific cities or areas with high demand for data services. These limited rollouts allow providers to gauge user response and gather real-world performance data;

- wider coverage: as infrastructure and technology mature, providers expand 5G coverage to additional cities and regions, eventually achieving nationwide coverage.

– Frequency spectrum allocation: governments and regulatory bodies allocate frequency spectrum for 5G networks. Different frequency bands have varying characteristics: lower bands provide broader coverage, while higher bands (like millimeter wave) offer faster speeds but have shorter ranges.

– Use case exploration: as 5G networks become more established, industries and developers explore new use cases and applications that leverage the capabilities of 5G technology. This includes areas such as healthcare, transportation, manufacturing, entertainment, smart cities and more.

– Integration of new services: telecommunication companies and service providers introduce new services and offerings that take advantage of 5G's capabilities. These could include ultra-high-definition streaming, augmented reality experiences, remote surgeries, smart city solutions and innovative IoT applications.

– Partnerships and collaboration: various stakeholders, including telecommunication providers, device manufacturers, governments and technology companies, collaborate to ensure a smooth transition to 5G. They work together to address technical challenges, regulatory requirements and the development of interoperable standards.

– Education and awareness: consumers, businesses and industries need to understand the benefits and potential of 5G. Education and awareness campaigns help users make informed decisions about adopting 5G-enabled devices and services.

– Addressing challenges: the adoption of 5G also comes with challenges such as infrastructure costs, regulatory approvals, addressing potential health concerns and ensuring cybersecurity and privacy in a more connected world.

The adoption of 5G involves a coordinated effort among various stakeholders, including telecommunication companies, technology providers, device manufacturers, regulatory bodies and consumers. It is a gradual process that starts with infrastructure development and device compatibility, leading to the deployment of networks and the exploration of innovative applications that leverage the capabilities of 5G technology.

11.10. Healthcare

Healthcare refers to the maintenance or improvement of an individual's physical, mental and emotional well-being through medical, preventive, diagnostic, therapeutic and support services. It encompasses a wide range of activities and professions aimed at promoting and maintaining health, preventing and treating illnesses, and enhancing the overall quality of life.

Key aspects of healthcare include:

– Medical treatment: healthcare is centered around medical treatment, which involves a spectrum of interventions aimed at diagnosing, managing and curing illnesses and injuries. Medical professionals, including doctors, surgeons, nurses and specialists, use a variety of techniques such as surgeries, medications, therapies and medical procedures to alleviate health issues. For instance, surgical procedures are performed to remove tumors, repair injuries, or transplant organs, while medications address infections, chronic diseases and pain management.

– Preventive care: an integral facet of healthcare is preventive care, which focuses on preemptively avoiding health problems. This encompasses regular health check-ups, screenings (such as mammograms and blood tests), vaccinations to immunize against diseases and lifestyle interventions such as promoting exercise, healthy diets and tobacco cessation. Preventive care plays a critical role in identifying risks early and minimizing the impact of potential health threats.

– Wellness and lifestyle management: healthcare extends beyond illness treatment to encompass education and support for maintaining a wholesome lifestyle. Healthcare professionals provide guidance on nutrition, exercise routines, stress management techniques and other habits that contribute to overall well-being. This proactive approach empowers individuals to make informed choices that foster their long-term health.

– Mental health support: recognizing the importance of mental well-being, healthcare includes services to address psychological issues. Mental health professionals, such as psychologists and psychiatrists, offer counseling, therapy and medication to manage conditions like anxiety, depression and bipolar disorder. Mental health support is vital for achieving a balanced state of emotional health.

– Emergency and urgent care: healthcare services encompass emergency and urgent care, providing immediate medical attention for severe or critical situations. Trauma centers, emergency rooms and urgent care clinics are equipped to handle accidents, injuries, heart attacks, strokes and other life-threatening conditions, ensuring prompt medical assistance when time is of the essence.

– Rehabilitation and recovery: following surgeries, injuries or chronic conditions, individuals often require rehabilitation and recovery services. Physical therapists, occupational therapists and speech therapists collaborate to aid patients in regaining mobility, functionality and independence. Rehabilitation programs involve exercises, therapies and techniques tailored to individual needs.

– Long-term care: healthcare addresses the needs of those requiring ongoing support due to chronic illnesses, disabilities or age-related issues. Long-term care encompasses a range of services, from nursing homes and assisted living facilities to home healthcare and hospice care. These services aim to maintain individuals' quality of life and ensure they receive proper care and attention.

– Healthcare systems: healthcare is organized into complex systems comprising hospitals, clinics, pharmacies, laboratories and administrative bodies. These systems work collaboratively to deliver comprehensive medical services. Hospitals provide various levels of care, from routine treatments to specialized surgeries. Clinics offer outpatient care, diagnostics and preventive services. Pharmacies dispense medications, and laboratories conduct tests for accurate diagnoses. Healthcare administration oversees operations and regulations within the industry.

– Healthcare technology: technological advancements play a pivotal role in modern healthcare. Medical devices, ranging from imaging machines to pacemakers, aid in diagnostics and treatments. Telemedicine allows remote patient consultations through video calls. Electronic health records (EHRs) streamline patient data management. Innovative treatments, such as gene therapies and targeted drugs, emerge from medical research and technological innovations, contributing to better healthcare outcomes.

– Research and development: healthcare is perpetually evolving due to ongoing research and development efforts. Medical researchers explore new treatments, medications and interventions to enhance medical understanding and address health challenges. Clinical trials evaluate the effectiveness and safety of new therapies, enabling medical advancements. Research leads to the discovery of groundbreaking treatments and methodologies that revolutionize patient care.

Healthcare encompasses a multifaceted approach to promoting and sustaining individual and community health. It encompasses a wide spectrum of services, technologies and systems that address not only physical health but also mental and emotional well-being. By integrating medical treatment, preventive care, wellness management and technological advancements, healthcare strives to enhance the overall quality of life and minimize the impact of health-related issues on individuals and society as a whole.

11.11. 5G technology's impact on healthcare: a comprehensive overview

5G technology, the fifth generation of cellular networks, is poised to revolutionize industries across the globe, and healthcare is no exception. With its unprecedented speed, low latency, high reliability and massive device connectivity, 5G holds the potential to transform how healthcare is delivered, accessed and experienced. This comprehensive overview delves into the multifaceted role of 5G in healthcare, exploring its applications, benefits, challenges and future prospects.

– Connected ambulance: enhancing emergency care connected ambulances are a compelling example of 5G's potential in healthcare. With real-time data transmission and high-quality video streaming, 5G enables paramedics to relay crucial patient information to hospitals while en route. Specialists can guide paramedics through complex procedures remotely, optimizing patient outcomes. The combination of 5G's low latency and high bandwidth is essential for split-second decision-making during emergencies.

– High-definition virtual consultations: revolutionizing telemedicine: High-definition virtual consultations powered by 5G redefine telemedicine. Patients can engage in two-way video consultations with healthcare professionals, offering initial screenings, routine check-ups and even visual diagnoses. 5G's mobility and reliability facilitate seamless interactions, reducing the need for physical visits, cutting costs and enhancing patient convenience.

– Remote patient monitoring and proactive healthcare management: remote patient monitoring leverages 5G's capabilities to collect and transmit patient data in real time. Wearables, sensors and e-health devices enable continuous monitoring, supporting proactive disease management. The high reliability and security of 5G networks ensure accurate data transmission, empowering patients and healthcare providers with actionable insights.

– Video-enabled medication adherence: enhancing compliance video-enabled medication adherence solutions leverage 5G to connect patients with pharmacists and caregivers via video calls. This technology ensures patients take medications correctly, benefiting the elderly and those with mental health conditions. 5G's high bandwidth and low latency improve patient compliance and reduce medication errors.

– Augmented reality and virtual reality for the visually impaired: enabling independence 5G-powered augmented reality (AR) and virtual reality (VR) solutions empower the visually impaired by providing real-time connections to advisors. These technologies assist individuals with tasks such as navigation and everyday activities, enhancing their independence and quality of life. 5G's low latency is vital for seamless interaction, ensuring a comfortable experience.

– Distraction and rehabilitative therapy: innovative patient care AR and VR for distraction and rehabilitative therapy transform patient experiences. By immersing patients in virtual environments, 5G-powered solutions alleviate anxiety during medical procedures and provide relief for conditions like phantom limb pain. The technology's low latency and high bandwidth enhance the effectiveness of therapeutic interventions.

– Remote expert collaboration in surgery: advancing surgical practices 5G-enabled remote expert collaboration in surgery revolutionizes surgical procedures. Surgeons can receive real-time guidance from specialists through AR/VR headsets, enhancing precision and outcomes. The technology's low latency, high bandwidth and reliability facilitate seamless communication and visualization, fostering interdisciplinary collaboration.

– AR and VR for training and education: fostering learning 5G-powered AR/VR for training and education redefine medical education. Medical students and trainees can engage in immersive learning experiences, practicing procedures and collaborating in virtual simulations. 5G's low latency and high bandwidth enhance the quality of training, preparing healthcare professionals for real-world scenarios.

– Real-time high-throughput computational processing: accelerating diagnostics real-time high-throughput computational processing fueled by 5G accelerates diagnostics and drug design. Medical images can be transmitted and analyzed in real time, aiding in timely diagnoses. In the pharmaceutical industry, molecular models can be processed in the cloud, enhancing drug discovery processes.

– Video analytics for behavioral recognition: enhancing patient safety video analytics for behavioral recognition in healthcare facilities use 5G's capabilities to detect anomalies and potential dangers. Smart cameras equipped with analytics identify unusual behaviors, falls or risks to patients. 5G's high bandwidth and low latency enable real-time processing, contributing to patient safety.

– Privacy and security considerations: safeguarding patient data while 5G offers remarkable advancements, privacy and security considerations are paramount. The increasing volume of sensitive patient data requires robust encryption, authentication and secure communication protocols. As healthcare embraces 5G, organizations must prioritize cybersecurity to protect patient confidentiality.

– Challenges and adoption barriers: the widespread adoption of 5G in healthcare faces challenges, including infrastructure development, cost considerations and regulatory compliance. Healthcare organizations must invest in upgrading networks, implementing security measures and ensuring compliance with healthcare regulations.

– Future prospects, beyond the horizon: the future of 5G in healthcare holds promise for even more innovative applications. From tele-surgery advancements to IoT-enabled healthcare devices, the healthcare landscape is poised for further transformation. As technology evolves, 5G's potential in healthcare will continue to expand, reshaping patient care, medical education and research. The advent of 5G technology has the potential to revolutionize the healthcare sector by enabling innovative solutions, enhancing patient care and transforming the way medical services are delivered. Here is an in-depth look at the role of 5G in the healthcare sector:

– Telemedicine and remote patient monitoring: 5G's high-speed, low-latency capabilities are poised to transform telemedicine and remote patient monitoring. Healthcare providers can deliver real-time video consultations with patients, allowing for accurate diagnosis and treatment recommendations. Additionally, remote monitoring of patients' vital signs and health data becomes more feasible and reliable with 5G, enabling proactive intervention and reducing hospital readmissions.

– Figure high-quality imaging and diagnostics: 5G's enhanced bandwidth and low latency are vital for transmitting large medical imaging files like MRI scans and CT scans. This enables healthcare professionals to collaborate on complex cases, make quicker diagnoses and provide more informed treatment plans, regardless of their physical locations.

– Surgical advancements: in surgical procedures, 5G's low latency is crucial for real-time communication between surgeons and robotic systems. This capability can lead to more precise and minimally invasive surgeries, with surgeons controlling robotic instruments remotely while receiving high-definition visual feedback.

– Emergency response: 5G facilitates quick communication and data transfer during emergency situations. Emergency medical services (EMS) can transmit patient data, medical history and real-time information from the field to the hospital, enabling healthcare providers to be prepared and make informed decisions before the patient arrives.

– IoT-enabled healthcare devices: the Internet of Things (IoT) combined with 5G allows for seamless connectivity of various healthcare devices. Wearable health trackers, smart medical devices and sensors can transmit data in real-time, providing healthcare professionals with comprehensive insights into patients' health statuses and enabling early intervention.

– Medical training and education: 5G enables high-quality, real-time video streaming, making it possible for medical students and professionals to participate in virtual training sessions, surgical demonstrations and educational seminars from remote locations. This democratizes medical education and fosters continuous learning.

– Drug development and clinical trials: the speed and capacity of 5G can accelerate the sharing of data between researchers and institutions involved in drug development and clinical trials. This can streamline the research process, facilitate data analysis and potentially expedite the discovery of new treatments.

– Elderly care and aging population: with an aging global population, 5G-powered solutions can enhance elderly care through remote monitoring, fall detection systems and medication management. Seniors can age in place with increased independence while staying connected to healthcare providers.

– Data analytics and AI: the rapid data transfer enabled by 5G supports the use of advanced data analytics and artificial intelligence (AI) in healthcare. This can lead to more accurate diagnoses, personalized treatment plans and predictive insights for disease prevention. The 5G technology holds immense potential to reshape the healthcare sector, offering faster communication, real-time data transmission and a foundation for advanced medical applications. By improving connectivity, reducing latency and enabling a wide array of innovative solutions, 5G has the capacity to revolutionize patient care, medical procedures and healthcare delivery as a whole.

11.12. Conclusion

5G technology's impact on healthcare is profound and multifaceted. From connected ambulances to advanced surgical collaboration, 5G is driving transformative changes in patient care, medical education and healthcare management. While challenges remain, the potential benefits far outweigh the obstacles. As 5G continues to evolve, healthcare stands on the brink of a new era, where technology enhances accessibility, quality and efficiency in delivering healthcare services to individuals worldwide.

In summary, the dawn of 5G technology heralds a new era of connectivity and innovation, promising to reshape our digital landscape in profound ways. With its unprecedented data speeds, low latency and capacity for massive device connectivity, 5G holds the key to unlocking a realm of possibilities previously beyond our reach. From real-time applications that blur the lines between physical and virtual realities to the seamless interconnectivity of the Internet of Things, the impact of 5G on industries, societies and individual lives is poised to be transformative.

However, as we embrace the promises of 5G, we must also navigate the challenges it presents. The need for extensive infrastructure upgrades, discussions about privacy and security, and concerns regarding potential health effects underscore the importance of approaching 5G deployment with careful consideration and thoughtful regulation. It is imperative that we strike a balance between harnessing its power and addressing its complexities to ensure a responsible and inclusive integration of 5G technology.

As we stand on the cusp of this technological revolution, the journey ahead will be marked by collaboration, adaptation and innovation. The potential of 5G to revolutionize industries, from healthcare to entertainment, and to create smarter cities and more connected communities is undeniable. By embracing this evolution with a clear understanding of its advantages and challenges, we can pave the way for a future where the capabilities of 5G technology empower us to build a more interconnected, efficient and inclusive world.

11.13. References

Bangerter, B., Talwar, S., Arefi, R., Stewart, K. (2014). Networks and devices for the 5G era. *IEEE Commun. Mag.*, 52, 90–96.

Bhushan, N., Li, J., Malladi, D., Gilmore, R., Brenner, D., Damnjanovic, A., Sukhavasi, T., Patel, C., Geirhofer, S. (2014). Network densification: The dominant theme for wireless evolution into 5G. *IEEE Commun. Mag.*, 52, 82–89.

Chih Lin, I., Rowell, C., Han, S., Xu, Z., Li, G., Pan, Z. (2014). Towards green and soft: A 5G perspective. *IEEE Commun. Mag.*, 52(2), 66–73.

Fallgren, M. and Timus, B. (2013). Scenarios, requirements and KPIs for 5G mobile and wireless systems. Document, ICT-317669-METIS/D1.1, METIS.

Fettweiss, G. and Alamouti, S. (2014). 5G: Personal mobile internet beyond what cellular did to telephony. *IEEE Commun. Mag.*, 52, 140–145.

Gani, A., Li, X., Yang, L., Zakaria, O., Anuar, N.B. (2009). Multi-bandwidth data path design for 5G wireless mobile internets. *WSEAS Trans. Info. Sci. Appl.*, 6(2), 159–168.

He, C. and Gitlin, R.D. (2016). Limiting performance of massive MIMO downlink cellular systems. In *2016 Information Theory and Applications Workshop*, La Jolla. IEEE.

Hong, S., Brand, J., Choi, J.I., Jain, M., Mehlman, J., Katti, S., Levis, P. (2014). Applications of self-interference cancellation in 5G and beyond. *IEEE Commun. Mag.*, 52, 114–121.

Janevski, T. (2009). 5G mobile phone concept. In *2009 6th IEEE Consumer Communications and Networking Conference*, Las Vegas. IEEE.

Ni, Y., Liang, J., Shi, X., Ban, D. (2019). Research on key technology in 5G mobile communication network. *2019 International Conference on Intelligent Transportation, Big Data & Smart City (ICITBS)*, Changsha. IEEE.

Panhwar, M.A., Sulleman Memon, M., Saddar, S., Rajput, U. (2017). 5G future technology: Research challenges for an emerging wireless networks. *Int. J. Comput. Sci. Netw. Security*, 17(12), 201–206.

Selinis, I., Katsaros, K., Allayioti, M., Vahid, S., Tafazolli, R. (2018). The race to 5G era; LTE and WI-FI. *IEEE Access*, 6, 56598–56636.

Sharma, P., Verma, M., Sundriyal, N., Chauhan, J. (2014). 5G mobile wireless technology. *Int. J. Res.*, 1(9), 631–634.

Turkiewicz, J.P. (2019). Optical transmission technologies for 5G networks. *21st International Conference on Transparent Optical Networks (ICTON)*, Angers. IEEE.

Won, S.H., Mueck, M., Frascolla, V., Kim, J., Destino, G., Pärssinen, A., Latva-aho, M., Korvala, A., Clemente, A., Kim, T. et al. (2017). Development of 5G CHAMPION testbeds for 5G services at the 2018 Winter Olympic Games. *IEEE Workshop on Signal Processing Advances in Wireless Communications* (SPAWC), Sapporo. IEEE.

Wu, Z., Wu, B., Su, Z., Zhang, X. (2018). Development challenges for 5G base station antennas. *2018 International Workshop on Antenna Technology (iWAT)*, Nanjing. IEEE.

Xu, J., Wang, J., Zhu, Y., Yang, Y., Zheng, X., Wang, S., Liu, L., Horne-man, K., Teng, Y. (2014). Cooperative distributed optimization for the hyper-dense small cell deployment. *IEEE Commun. Mag.*, 52, 61–67.

Yuk, K., Branner, G.R., Cui, C. (2017). Future directions for GaN in 5G and satellite communications. *2017 IEEE 60th International Midwest Symposium on Circuits and Systems (MWSCAS)*, Boston. IEEE.

List of Authors

Manpreet Kaur AIDEN
Sharda University
Knowledge Park III
Greater Noida
India

Sai AYUSH
Department of ECE
Acharya Institute of Technology
Bangalore
India

Prasenjit CHATTERJEE
MCKV Institute of Engineering
West Bengal
India

Sonia CHHABRA
Sharda University
Knowledge Park III
Greater Noida
India

Mansi CHITGOPEKAR
Amity University
Mumbai
India

Varalakshmi DANDU
JNTUA School of Management
Studies
India

Deepa DAS
Shri Ramdeobaba College of
Engineering and Management
Nagpur
India

Rohit DEY
Institute of Nursing Science
Agartala
India

Rakesh Kumar DIXIT
GL Bajaj Institute of Management
Greater Noida
India

Obiora Reginald EJINAKA
Office of Deputy Provost Academics
Federal School of Medical
Laboratory Science
Jos
Nigeria

Nkereuwem Sunday ETUKUDOH
Office of Deputy Provost Academics
Federal School of Medical
Laboratory Science
Jos
Nigeria

Sai Sreeram GADDE
Department of ECE
Acharya Institute of Technology
Bangalore
India

Manthan GHOSH
G H Raisoni College of Engineering
Nagpur
India

Bhawna KAUSHIK
GL Bajaj Institute of Management
Greater Noida
India

Ranjan K. MOHAPATRA
Department of Chemistry
Government College of Engineering
Keonjhar
Odisha
India

Abdul Raffie NAIK
Acharya Institute of Technology
Bangalore
India

Uchejeso Mark OBETA
Department of Medical Laboratory
Management
Federal School of Medical
Laboratory Science
Jos
Nigeria

Amaechi Eze ODONO
Department of Immunology/Virology
Federal School of Medical
Laboratory Science
Jos
Nigeria

Srinivasa Murthy OMKAR
Department of ECE
Acharya Institute of Technology
Bangalore
India

Madhumita PAL
Department of Electrical Engineering
Government College of Engineering
Keonjhar
and
Department of Electronics and
Communication
C. V. Raman Global University
Bhubaneswar
Odisha
India

Bhanudas Suresh PANCHBHAI
Department of Computer Science
R. C. Patel Arts Commerce and
Science College
Maharashtra
India

Ganapati PANDA
Department of Electronics
and Communication
C. V. Raman Global University
Bhubaneswar
Odisha
India

Smita PARIJA
Department of Electronics
and Communication
C. V. Raman Global University
Bhubaneswar
Odisha
India

Varsha Makarand PATHAK
Department of Computer Application
KCE's Institute of Management and
Research
Maharashtra
3ywIndia

Devasis PRADHAN
Acharya Institute of Technology
Bengaluru
India

RAJESWARI
Department of ECE
Acharya Institute of Technology
Bangalore
India

Shweta Mayor SABBHARWAL
Galgotias University
Greater Noida
India

Prasanna Kumar SAHU
NIT Rourkela
Odisha
India

Mayank SAINI
GL Bajaj Institute of Management
Greater Noida
India

Pushpendra Pal SINGH
GL Bajaj Institute of Management
Greater Noida
India

Nitish SINHA
Tripura University
Agartala
India

Siddabassappa Manjunath SUJAN
Department of ECE
Acharya Institute of Technology
Bangalore
India

Shivarudraiah SUMALATHA
Department of ECE
Acharya Institute of Technology
Bangalore
India

Hla Myo TUN
Yangon Technological University
(YTU)
Myanmar

Mahimna VYAS
University of Bolton
UK

Index

A, B

C, D

E, F

G, I

K, L

M, N

P, R

S, T, V

Other titles from

ISTE

in

Computer Engineering

2024

CHAKRABORTY Rajdeep, GHOSH Anupam, KUMAR MANDAL Jyotsna, CHOUDHURY TANUPRIYA, CHATTERJEE Prasenjit
Smart Edge Computing: An Operation Research Perspective
(International Perspectives in Decision Analytics and Operations Research Set – Volume 2)

2023

CHOUDHURY Tanupriya, KHANNA Abhirup, CHATTERJEE Prasenjit, UM Jung-Sup, BHATTACHARYA Abhishek
Blockchain Applications in Healthcare: Innovations and Practices
(International Perspectives in Decision Analytics and Operations Research Set – Volume 1)

PAI G A Vijayalakshmi
A Textbook of Data Structures and Algorithms 1: Mastering Linear Data Structures
A Textbook of Data Structures and Algorithms 2: Mastering Nonlinear Data Structures
A Textbook of Data Structures and Algorithms 3: Mastering Advanced Data Structures and Algorithm Design Strategies

2022

HOMÈS Bernard
Advanced Testing of Systems-of-Systems 1: Theoretical Aspects
Advanced Testing of Systems-of-Systems 2: Practical Aspects

MEHTA Shikha, TIWARI Sanju, SIARRY Patrick, JABBAR M.A.
Tools, Languages, Methodologies for Representing Semantics on the Web of Things

SIDHOM Sahbi, KADDOUR Amira
Systems and Uses of Digital Sciences for Knowledge Organization (Digital Tools and Uses Set – Volume 9)

ZAIDOUN Ameur Salem
Computer Science Security: Concepts and Tools

2021

DELHAYE Jean-Loïc
Inside the World of Computing: Technologies, Uses, Challenges

HARDIN Thérèse, JAUME Mathieu, PESSAUX François,
VIGUIÉ DONZEAU-GOUGE Véronique
Concepts and Semantics of Programming Languages 1: A Semantical Approach with OCaml and Python
Concepts and Semantics of Programming Languages 2: Modular and Object-oriented Constructs with OCaml, Python, C++, Ada and Java

MKADMI Abderrazak
Archives in The Digital Age: Preservation and the Right to be Forgotten (Digital Tools and Uses Set – Volume 8)

TOKLU Yusuf Cengiz, BEKDAS Gebrail, NIGDELI Sinan Melih
Metaheuristics for Structural Design and Analysis (Optimization Heuristics Set – Volume 3)

2020

DARCHE Philippe
Microprocessor 1: Prolegomenes – Calculation and Storage Functions – Models of Computation and Computer Architecture
Microprocessor 2: Core Concepts – Communication in a Digital System
Microprocessor 3: Core Concepts – Hardware Aspects
Microprocessor 4: Core Concepts – Software Aspects
Microprocessor 5: Software and Hardware Aspects of Development, Debugging and Testing – The Microcomputer

DUVAUT Patrick, DALLOZ Xavier, MENGA David, KOEHL François, CHRIQUI Vidal, BRILL Joerg
Internet of Augmented Me, I.AM: Empowering Innovation for a New Sustainable Future

LAFFLY Dominique
TORUS 1 – Toward an Open Resource Using Services: Cloud Computing for Environmental Data
TORUS 2 – Toward an Open Resource Using Services: Cloud Computing for Environmental Data
TORUS 3 – Toward an Open Resource Using Services: Cloud Computing for Environmental Data

LAURENT Anne, LAURENT Dominique, MADERA Cédrine
Data Lakes
(Databases and Big Data Set – Volume 2)

OULHADJ Hamouche, DAACHI Boubaker, MENASRI Riad
Metaheuristics for Robotics
(Optimization Heuristics Set – Volume 2)

SADIQUI Ali
Computer Network Security

VENTRE Daniel
Artificial Intelligence, Cybersecurity and Cyber Defense

2019

BESBES Walid, DHOUIB Diala, WASSAN Niaz, MARREKCHI Emna
Solving Transport Problems: Towards Green Logistics

CLERC Maurice
Iterative Optimizers: Difficulty Measures and Benchmarks

GHLALA Riadh
Analytic SQL in SQL Server 2014/2016

TOUNSI Wiem
Cyber-Vigilance and Digital Trust: Cyber Security in the Era of Cloud Computing and IoT

2018

ANDRO Mathieu
Digital Libraries and Crowdsourcing
(Digital Tools and Uses Set – Volume 5)

ARNALDI Bruno, GUITTON Pascal, MOREAU Guillaume
Virtual Reality and Augmented Reality: Myths and Realities

CARDON Alain
Beyond Artificial Intelligence: From Human Consciousness to Artificial Consciousness

HOMAYOUNI S. Mahdi, FONTES Dalila B.M.M.
Metaheuristics for Maritime Operations
(Optimization Heuristics Set – Volume 1)

JEANSOULIN Robert
JavaScript and Open Data

PIVERT Olivier
NoSQL Data Models: Trends and Challenges
(Databases and Big Data Set – Volume 1)

SEDKAOUI Soraya
Data Analytics and Big Data

SALEH Imad, AMMI Mehdi, SZONIECKY Samuel
Challenges of the Internet of Things: Technology, Use, Ethics
(Digital Tools and Uses Set – Volume 7)

SZONIECKY Samuel
Ecosystems Knowledge: Modeling and Analysis Method for Information and Communication
(Digital Tools and Uses Set – Volume 6)

2017

BENMAMMAR Badr
Concurrent, Real-Time and Distributed Programming in Java: Threads, RTSJ and RMI

BOUHAÏ Nasreddine, SALEH Imad
Internet of Things: Evolutions and Innovations
(Digital Tools and Uses Set – Volume 4)

HÉLIODORE Frédéric, NAKIB Amir, ISMAIL Boussaad, OUCHRAA Salma, SCHMITT Laurent
Metaheuristics for Intelligent Electrical Networks
(Metaheuristics Set – Volume 10)

MA Haiping, SIMON Dan
Evolutionary Computation with Biogeography-based Optimization
(Metaheuristics Set – Volume 8)

PÉTROWSKI Alain, BEN-HAMIDA Sana
Evolutionary Algorithms
(Metaheuristics Set – Volume 9)

PAI G A Vijayalakshmi
Metaheuristics for Portfolio Optimization
(Metaheuristics Set – Volume 11)

REYES-GARCIA Everardo
The Image-Interface: Graphical Supports for Visual Information
(Digital Tools and Uses – Volume 3)

REYES-GARCIA Everardo, BOUHAÏ Nasreddine
Designing Interactive Hypermedia Systems
(Digital Tools and Uses – Volume 2)

SZONIECKY Samuel, BOUHAÏ Nasreddine
Collective Intelligence and Digital Archives: Towards Knowledge Ecosystems
(Digital Tools and Uses Set – Volume 1)

2016

BLUM Christian, FESTA Paola
Metaheuristics for String Problems in Bio-informatics
(Metaheuristics Set – Volume 6)

DEROUSSI Laurent
Metaheuristics for Logistics
(Metaheuristics Set – Volume 4)

DHAENENS Clarisse, JOURDAN Laetitia
Metaheuristics for Big Data
(Metaheuristics Set – Volume 5)

LABADIE Nacima, PRINS Christian, PRODHON Caroline
Metaheuristics for Vehicle Routing Problems
(Metaheuristics Set – Volume 3)

LEROY Laure
Eyestrain Reduction in Stereoscopy

LUTTON Evelyne, PERROT Nathalie, TONDA Albert
Evolutionary Algorithms for Food Science and Technology
(Metaheuristics Set – Volume 7)

MAGOULÈS Frédéric, ZHAO Hai-Xiang
Data Mining and Machine Learning in Building Energy Analysis

RIGO Michel
Advanced Graph Theory and Combinatorics

ZELM Martin, DOUMEINGTS Guy, MENDONÇA Joao Pedro
Enterprise Interoperability: in the Digitized and Networked Factory of the Future

2015

BARBIER Franck, RECOUSSINE Jean-Luc
COBOL Software Modernization: From Principles to Implementation with the BLU AGE® Method

CHEN Ken
Performance Evaluation by Simulation and Analysis with Applications to Computer Networks

CLERC Maurice
Guided Randomness in Optimization
(Metaheuristics Set – Volume 1)

DURAND Nicolas, GIANAZZA David, GOTTELAND Jean-Baptiste, ALLIOT Jean-Marc
Metaheuristics for Air Traffic Management
(Metaheuristics Set – Volume 2)

MAGOULÈS Frédéric, ROUX François-Xavier, HOUZEAUX Guillaume
Parallel Scientific Computing

MUNEESAWANG Paisarn, YAMMEN Suchart
Visual Inspection Technology in the Hard Disk Drive Industry

2014

BOULANGER Jean-Louis
Formal Methods Applied to Industrial Complex Systems
Formal Methods Applied to Complex Systems: Implementation of the B Method

EXPOSITO Ernesto, DIOP Codé
Smart SOA Platforms in Cloud Computing Architectures

GARDI Frédéric, BENOIST Thierry, DARLAY Julien, ESTELLON Bertrand, MEGEL Romain
Mathematical Programming Solver based on Local Search

KRICHEN Saoussen, CHAOUACHI Jouhaina
Graph-related Optimization and Decision Support Systems

LARRIEU Nicolas, VARET Antoine
Rapid Prototyping of Software for Avionics Systems: Model-oriented Approaches for Complex Systems Certification

LAURAS Matthieu, ZELM Martin, ARCHIMÈDE Bernard, BÉNABEN Frédérick DOUMEINGTS Guy
Enterprise Interoperability: Interoperability for Agility, Resilience and Plasticity of Collaborations

OUSSALAH Mourad Chabane
Software Architecture 1
Software Architecture 2

PASCHOS Vangelis Th
Combinatorial Optimization – 3-volume series, 2nd Edition
Concepts of Combinatorial Optimization – Volume 1, 2nd Edition
Problems and New Approaches – Volume 2, 2nd Edition
Applications of Combinatorial Optimization – Volume 3, 2nd Edition

QUESNEL Flavien
Scheduling of Large-scale Virtualized Infrastructures: Toward Cooperative Management

RIGO Michel
Formal Languages, Automata and Numeration Systems 1: Introduction to Combinatorics on Words
Formal Languages, Automata and Numeration Systems 2: Applications to Recognizability and Decidability

SAINT-DIZIER Patrick
Musical Rhetoric: Foundations and Annotation Schemes

TOUATI Sid, DUPONT DE DINECHIN Benoit
Advanced Backend Optimization

2013

ANDRÉ Etienne, SOULAT Romain
The Inverse Method: Parametric Verification of Real-time Embedded Systems

BOULANGER Jean-Louis
Safety Management for Software-based Equipment

DELAHAYE Daniel, PUECHMOREL Stéphane
Modeling and Optimization of Air Traffic

FRANCOPOULO Gil
LMF — Lexical Markup Framework

GHEDIRA Khaled
Constraint Satisfaction Problems: CSP Formalisms and Techniques

GOVAERT Gérard, NADIF Mohamed
Co-Clustering: Models, Algorithms and Applications

LANDRAGIN Frédérick
Man–Machine Dialogue: Design and Challenges

LUCAS Laurent, LOSCOS Céline, REMION Yannick
3D Video: Models, From Capture to Diffusion

ROCHANGE Christine, UHRIG Sascha, SAINRAT Pascal
Time-Predictable Architectures

WAHBI Mohamed
Algorithms and Ordering Heuristics for Distributed Constraint Satisfaction Problems

ZELM Martin, VAN SINDEREN Marten, FERRAIRA PIRES Luis, DOUMEINGTS Guy
Enterprise Interoperability: Research and Applications in the Service-oriented Ecosystem

2012

ARBOLEDA Hugo, ROYER Jean-Claude
Model-Driven and Software Product Line Engineering

BLANCHET Gérard, DUPOUY Bertrand
Computer Architecture

BOULANGER Jean-Louis
Industrial Use of Formal Methods: Formal Verification
Formal Method: Industrial Use from Model to the Code

CALVARY Gaëlle, DELOT Thierry, SEDES Florence, TIGLI Jean-Yves
Computer Science and Ambient Intelligence

MAHOUT Vincent
Assembly Language Programming: ARM Cortex-M3 2.0: Organization, Innovation and Territory

MARLET Renaud
Program Specialization

SOTO Maria, SEVAUX Marc, ROSSI André, LAURENT Johann
Memory Allocation Problems in Embedded Systems: Optimization Methods

2011

BICHOT Charles-Edmond, SIARRY Patrick
Graph Partitioning

BOULANGER Jean-Louis
Static Analysis of Software: The Abstract Interpretation

CAFERRA Ricardo
Logic for Computer Science and Artificial Intelligence

HOMÈS Bernard
Fundamentals of Software Testing

KORDON Fabrice, HADDAD Serge, PAUTET Laurent, PETRUCCI Laure
Distributed Systems: Design and Algorithms
Models and Analysis in Distributed Systems

LORCA Xavier
Tree-based Graph Partitioning Constraint

RIDHA MAHJOUB A.
Progress in Combinatorial Optimization: ISCO2010

TRUCHET Charlotte, ASSAYAG Gerard
Constraint Programming in Music

VICAT-BLANC PRIMET Pascale *et al.*
Computing Networks: From Cluster to Cloud Computing

2010

AUBRUN Christophe, SIMON Daniel, SONG Ye-Qiong
Co-design Approaches for Dependable Networked Control Systems

AUDIBERT Pierre
Mathematics for Informatics and Computer Science

BABAU Jean-Philippe, BLAY-FORNARINO Mireille, CHAMPEAU Joël, ROBERT Sylvain, SABETTA Antonino
Model Driven Engineering for Distributed Real-Time Embedded Systems: MARTE modeling, model transformations and their usages

BOULANGER Jean-Louis
Safety of Computer Architectures

BUFFET OLIVIER, Sigaud OLIVIER
Markov Decision Processes in Artificial Intelligence

MONMARCHÉ Nicolas, GUINAND Frédérick, SIARRY Patrick
Artificial Ants

PANETTO Hervé, BOUDJLIDA Nacer
Interoperability for Enterprise Software and Applications 2010

SOLNON Christine
Ant Colony Optimization and Constraint Programming

2009

FOURNIER Jean-Claude
Graph Theory and Applications: with exercises and problems

GUÉDON Jeanpierre
The Mojette Transform: Theory and Applications

JARD Claude, ROUX Olivier H.
Communicating Embedded Systems: Software and Design

LECOUTRE Christophe
Constraint Networks: Targeting Simplicity for Techniques and Algorithms

2008

BANÂTRE Michel, MARRON Pedro Jose, OLLERO Anibal, WOLITZ Adam
Cooperating Embedded Systems and Wireless Sensor Networks

MERZ Stephan, NAVET Nicolas
Modeling and Verification of Real-time Systems: Formalisms and Software Tools

PASCHOS Vangelis Th
Combinatorial Optimization and Theoretical Computer Science: Interfaces and Perspectives

WALDNER Jean-Baptiste
Nanocomputers and Swarm Intelligence

2007

BENHAMOU Frédéric, JUSSIEN Narendra, O'SULLIVAN Barry
Trends in Constraint Programming

JUSSIEN Narendra
A to Z of Sudoku

2006

BABAU Jean-Philippe, CHAMPEAU Joël, GÉRARD Sébastien
From MDD Concepts to Experiments and Illustrations – DRES 2006

HABRIAS Henri, FRAPPIER Marc
Software Specification Methods: An Overview Using a Case Study

MURAT Cécile, PASCHOS Vangelis Th
Probabilistic Combinatorial Optimization on Graphs

PANETTO Hervé, BOUDJLIDA Nacer
Interoperability for Enterprise Software and Applications 2006: IFAC-IFIP I-ESA'2006

2005

GÉRARD Sébastien, BABAU Jean-Philippe, CHAMPEAU Joël
Model Driven Engineering for Distributed Real Time Embedded Systems

PANETTO Hervé
Interoperability of Enterprise Software and Applications 2005

Printed and bound by CPI Group (UK) Ltd, Croydon, CR0 4YY

16/09/2026

14963077-0004